Praise for *Give Birth Lik...*

'A radical new book.' ***The S...***

'A manifesto for the birthing woman.' *The Economist*

'Hill's book leaves the reader not just well-informed,
but with a renewed sense of pride in the power of the
female body.' **Victoria Smith, author of *Hags***

'Clear, compelling and convincing ... Milli Hill's exploration of
childbirth as central feminist issue is a must-read.' **Soraya Chemaly**

'Milli gets it. Birth matters to women, to
society, birth *is* a *feminist* issue.'
**Sheena Byrom OBE**

'This is not a book just for expectant mums. Everyone should read
it, especially doctors, nurses, midwives, partners and grandparents.
The world has changed and this awesome book connects the dots
in a way that can change minds and improve outcomes. Bravo!'
**Tina Cassidy, author of *Birth: A History***

'A rallying cry for women everywhere ... everyone
should read this book and look at childbirth through
a feminist lens.' **Ricki Lake, Producer and Abby
Epstein, Director: *The Business of Being Born***

'So extraordinary. It's transformed my
perspective of birth and labour considerably ... a
seminal work.' **The Grand Thunk Podcast**

'In case anyone is uncertain about what you're "allowed" to
do when giving birth, Hill spells it out: stop asking for permission,
recognize that your experience matters – quite a bit – and
demand respect. Hill joins the chorus with a loud call to action
for feminists: this is your issue, too.' **Jennifer Block, journalist
and author of *Pushed* and *Everything Below the Waist***

**Milli Hill** is a writer, feminist and freelance journalist with a passion for reframing the narrative around women's bodies. She is the author of the bestselling *Positive Birth Book* and *My Period*. From 2012 to 2021 she founded and ran the Positive Birth Movement, a global network of antenatal discussion groups aimed at improving birth and giving women better access to support and information.

She has written for many publications including the *Telegraph, Daily Mail, Guardian, Independent* and *Mother&Baby*. She has appeared on BBC Radio 4, BBC Radio 2, BBC 5 Live, TalkRadio, LBC as well as many leading podcasts. She lives in Somerset with her partner and three children.

# Give Birth Like a Feminist

### Your Body. Your Baby. Your Choices.

## Milli Hill

ONE PLACE. MANY STORIES

HQ
An imprint of HarperCollins*Publishers* Ltd
1 London Bridge Street
London SE1 9GF

www.harpercollins.co.uk

HarperCollins*Publishers*
Macken House, 39/40 Mayor Street Upper,
Dublin 1, D01 C9W8, Ireland

This edition 2023

1
First published in Great Britain by
HQ, an imprint of HarperCollins*Publishers* Ltd 2019

ISBN: 978-0-00-831313-5

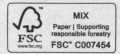

This book is produced from independently certified FSC™ paper
to ensure responsible forest management.

For more information visit: www.harpercollins.co.uk/green

This book is set in Minion by Type-it AS, Norway

Printed and Bound in the UK using 100% Renewable Electricity at
CPI Group (UK) Ltd, Croydon, CR0 4YY

# Contents

**Chapter 7**

**Chapter 8**

# Introduction

*Birth is a feminist issue. And it's the feminist issue nobody's talking about. This book aims to start that conversation.*

As I've gone through the process of writing this book, I've had a few moments where I've wondered, why me? My inner critic (don't try to tell me you haven't got one of those) has said to me, 'Milli? Do you really want to open this particular can of worms? As if talking about childbirth wasn't treacherous enough, now you want to drop the F-bomb?! Are you nuts? That is literally the worst combination of topics. You are going to get burned at the stake – well, metaphorically speaking, at least.' My inner critic is such a gas.

It's true, it's not always easy to talk about childbirth, and it's not always easy to raise feminist issues. People can even argue about what feminism actually is, but to me it's simple: feminism just means noticing when women are getting a raw deal, and taking action. And this is where the problem lies with childbirth. Not enough people are noticing that women are getting a raw deal, and not enough people are taking action. We've become blinkered to the massive imbalance of power in the birth room, and somehow come to accept that birth is inherently unpleasant and undignified, or even traumatic, degrading and violating. 'That's just how it is!' Well I want this book to tell you it doesn't have to be that way, and as feminists we must no longer tolerate this state of affairs.

Feminism doesn't have to be complicated, and it doesn't have to be exclusive. Giving birth like a feminist doesn't mean giving birth a certain way, just as doing anything else – career, relationships, parenting – 'like a feminist' doesn't require a one-size-fits-all approach. You can give birth like a feminist in any setting and in any way, from elective caesarean in a private hospital to freebirth in the ocean. All that's required is that you have somehow moved from a passive place where you view birth as something that happens to you and over which you have no control, to a place of understanding that you may get a raw deal in this experience if you don't wake up and get yourself into the driving seat. Essentially: take charge, take control, and make conscious choices.

When I speak at mainstream maternity events, I am often shocked by the fact that telling women and their partners that they have rights and choices in the birth room so often seems to come as a revelation. Many people have no sense of themselves as autonomous or powerful in their labour and birth, nor do they feel that there is anything they can do or not do to influence the way their birth unfolds. They are often misinformed and, to compound this, their belief that they have little or no agency then prevents them from seeking out much information. What is the point in learning about your options against a backdrop in which the phrase 'not allowed' is used with such alarming frequency? Most pregnant couples believe that the majority of choices are out of their hands. In practical terms this means that, on a daily basis, fingers enter the vaginas of women who do not know they can decline. How can this be acceptable? Even the most progressive of maternity conversations emphasises 'informed consent', with the unspoken assumption that *consent*, not 'decision making', or possibly even 'informed refusal', is the goal. Maternity professionals will speak of how they 'consent' women – using it as a verb, 'I am just going to go and *consent* her', as if the professional is the active one in the exchange and the women herself is passive. It's time to challenge a system that perpetuates this myth of unquestioning co-operation and female powerlessness.

When you raise a complaint about a female experience, you quite often get quickly reminded of how unusual, niche or rare the problem is, and just how good so many women have it. This focus-shifting is epitomised so well by the hashtag #notallmen – used to remind women just how many good, well-rounded men there are in the world when they try to highlight any issue from mansplaining to rape. '#notallmen are rapists. #notallmen have sexist attitudes. #notallmen beat their wives, remember!' Hang on, the women say, we don't want to talk about the large percentage of wonderful men who respect women – we want to talk about the other bunch, who don't. But in the diversion, the point has already been diluted, making the aggressor seem like the victim in the process. This diversionary tactic happens in conversations about birth, too. Attempts to complain about anything from lack of consent, to women not being properly listened to in labour, to institutionalised misogyny and racism in maternity care, are so often met with protests from health workers of 'It's not like that where I work!' or 'Not all midwives/obstetricians are like that, it's important not to make sweeping statements', etc. So, before we get started on our journey through this book, I want to stress that my focus throughout is not on individuals, but on the systems in which they operate. Maternity care is a system that needs to be challenged, built by and within another system that needs to be challenged – patriarchy. Please don't divert attention from this vital issue if you feel that you personally are working in a way that fully respects women as autonomous, or if you received gold-standard care in your own pregnancy. This is indeed wonderful, but it's not really what we are all here to talk about.

Likewise, there can sometimes be protests that we should be doing more to celebrate the wonderful men – and in the same way the wonderful maternity care providers – who are 'getting it right'. It's true, there are some brilliant midwives, doctors, obstetric units and organisations out there who are providing the most fantastic, refreshing, woman-centred, personalised maternity care – and yes, praise is a good thing, and yes, some of them are in this book. But do we really need to repeatedly celebrate those who are simply providing what women need and deserve? Do men who treat women with respect need a great big pat on the back? No – they are simply behaving normally, with the required, standard levels of kindness and compassion. There should not have to be medals for this, and for the same reasons I have not devoted endless pages of this book to good, decent, rights-based maternity care. Listening to women, caring for them as individuals, and respecting them as the key decision maker in the birth room should cease to be seen as a shining beacon in the darkness and start to be viewed as the baseline norm.

Currently, we are not getting birth right. This matters primarily because birth is a key human experience that will be remembered in great detail by a woman, and her partner, for the rest of their lives. In this book I have tried to ask some difficult questions about the kind of births women are currently experiencing vs. the kind of births that may be possible or desired. These are not easy conversations to have, not least because all women are different and will want and prioritise different things. Added to this, there is a weight of emotion brought to the discussion by those women who have already given birth and had traumatic or disempowering experiences. In spite of the complexity of the topic and the difficult feelings that discussing it evokes, I sincerely hope that this book will pull women together to work on this problem by truly listening to each other and in the true feminist spirit of solidarity. We owe it to those who are yet to give birth to ensure that we all collectively approve of the direction that the birth experience is taking.

Intervention rates in childbirth are rising rapidly, and we should all be concerned about this. This is not just my personal viewpoint. Leading bodies such as the World Health Organisation have expressed concern that the medicalisation of childbirth, with its focus on how to monitor, measure and control birth, has left the question of how women actually *feel* about their births completely off the agenda, potentially robbing them of a life-enhancing experience. [1]

The world's most prestigious medical journal, *The Lancet*, has drawn attention to the 'too much too soon' approach to birth, most often found in high-income countries, in which treatments that were originally designed to manage complications are now overused, missing an opportunity for women to feel strong and capable.[2] You will notice that in this book I have given plenty of attention to the issues around 'natural' or 'physiological' birth, because I do feel that this is a key topic for feminist focus. In writing about natural birth, I have often had the sense that I am 'championing the underdog'. Because we have to accept that, currently, natural birth – in which a woman has a baby without any pharmacological input such as induction, augmentation or drugs to expel the placenta – is very rare. Rarer still are what I call 'hands-off' births, in which women, rather than being 'managed', rely on their own instinct, follow their body's lead, and are not guided into certain positions or told when and how to push. Women who have their baby in this way, feeling totally confident in the loving support (and, if necessary, medical help) that they know is in place in the background, but left to give birth entirely under their own steam, will most often talk of the experience in evangelical terms, as life-changing moments in which they felt sexual, sensual, strong, vital and powerful. You can't help but wonder when you hear their stories how much the world might change if more women were getting this transformative power boost as they crossed the threshold to motherhood. Instead, it's becoming much more 'normal' to have a birth in which you feel unsupported, disempowered and traumatised. I therefore feel it's vital that we have a conversation about the value to women of this type of 'straightforward', 'physiological' or 'natural' type of birth experience, which is currently on the brink of extinction.

We also need to talk about those women who don't want or cannot have straightforward vaginal births. There is literally not one single birth scenario in which increasing empathy for the woman, listening to her voice, respecting her decisions, and honouring that this is an extraordinary day in her life will not be valid. There is literally not one single type of birth that we cannot improve upon. The best way to find out more about this is again to *listen to women*. I learned so much about what women want in birth from talking to those who have experienced caesarean, and in particular, caesarean under general anaesthetic – often the most difficult birth experience to process and recover from. From them I learned that the smallest of gestures can make the biggest and most life-changing differences. Taking a few moments to photograph the newborn on their mother's chest, for example, even if she is still unconscious, will create something she will treasure for a lifetime, a tangible antidote to her trauma. Women repeat again and again how much it means to them to know that their hands were among the first to touch their baby, even if they were not 'there' to experience it. Every small gesture matters, and we can always do better.

Two radical ideas underpin this book. Firstly, birth is a really important experience in a woman's life and it's time to stop telling women that it's 'just one day' in which they 'leave their dignity at the door' because a 'healthy baby is all that matters'. These are old-fashioned ideas, riddled with disrespect for women, for their autonomy, and for their feelings as sentient humans, that have no place in the twenty-first century. This book will try to unpick these ideas by looking at some of the history of birth, at various feminist perspectives, at the links between birth, female sexuality and power, and at the current culture of fear and disempowerment that continues to prop up these faded ideologies. Simultaneously, the book will try to replace these outdated perspectives with new considerations of women's rights in childbirth, their bodily integrity, in particular through the lens of #metoo, and take a fresh look at what we might find, both literally and figuratively, in a birth room built with women's needs in mind.

The second radical suggestion that this book will make is that pregnant women should be elevated to the role of key decision maker and most powerful person in the birth room. I can tell you from a decade of talking to women about their maternity care that, while there may be frequent reassurances that this is already the case, in reality it tends to make people uneasy. We see this most clearly when women try to go against the flow, birth outside of guidelines or refuse to consent to or accept the standard protocol or approach. These women, and often too, the midwives or doulas who support their choice 'no matter what', will often meet huge resistance, and risk sanctions or even punishment, as we will see in several stories in this book. We need a shift in consciousness, that moves to trusting women to make the right choices for themselves and for their baby. We need an acceptance that the image of a wayward, misinformed, irresponsible or even 'mad' woman, who does not have the best interests of her baby at heart, is a damaging and misogynist stereotype, used to justify the control of women, and rarely to be found in reality.

In this book you will find several references to 'freebirth' – where women choose not to have any medical professionals attend them but simply give birth by themselves. I have to be honest with you and say that I personally would never choose to birth without medical back-up. However, I totally and utterly support another woman's decision to make this choice. Do you? Because I believe that the key to birth freedom, for all of us, lies in supporting women in choices that we would not make ourselves, or even choices that we just feel are plain 'wrong'. We need to trust women. Ironically, if we manage to move to this place, we may suddenly find that the numbers of women who wish to freebirth or birth outside the system, begins to decline. Increasing numbers of women, quite understandably, don't want to birth in a system that doesn't listen to them, respect them or trust them.

Whether you are reading this book as a pregnant woman, a health care provider, or just as a person who cares about women's issues, I hope it switches on a light for you. First and foremost I hope that birth is suddenly illuminated as a feminist issue for you in a way that, perhaps, it never has been before. I hope it gets you thinking about the ways in which birth matters, about women's power, agency and autonomy in birth and about what we could be doing differently or better. I hope you are excited or inspired by some of the things you read in these pages and, equally, I am sure that there will be parts that you fervently disagree with, that are hard to hear, or that even make you angry. That's OK. As I keep telling my adorable inner critic, there will be many different reactions to this book, but ultimately all of them, 'good' and 'bad', will be much-needed voices, adding to the dialogue about birth as a feminist issue and moving it forwards. And this is essential if we wish to create a future in which women get the positive experiences of birth that they so desperately want, the medical help they truly need, and the power, respect and autonomy they so absolutely deserve. Let's start the conversation.

# Chapter 1
# 'Am I Allowed?': The Birth Room Power Imbalance

*The most common way people give up their power is by thinking they don't have any.*

Alice Walker[1]

The year is 1975. A woman in a hospital nightgown, shaky on her feet, is wandering the corridor outside the labour ward, using the wall to support her. It's 3 a.m. She is looking for something she has lost: her baby.

On the previous day several things happened to her that were 'routine'. When I say 'routine', what I really mean is that nobody asked her permission. She was induced because she was past her due date. Her pubic hair was shaved off. She was given an enema. The opioid pethidine was injected into her thigh shortly before delivery.

And her perfectly healthy baby was given to her and her husband to hold for a while, before being taken off to the hospital nursery for the night. She did not actively consent to any of this. It was just 'how it was done'.

Ushered back to bed by the stern but kindly matron, my mother never questioned her experiences of birth until, several decades later, she began to hear a new narrative from the baby they had taken to the nursery – me. In the midst of my own pregnancy journeys, I started to ask questions. 'How far past your due date were you?' 'Why did they shave women – was there any evidence to support this practice?' 'Did you ask for the pethidine?', 'Did they give me formula in the nursery?'

'I don't know. You didn't really ask questions then.'

'Why didn't you just tell them you wanted to keep your baby with you?'

'Well . . . they just didn't let you do that I suppose. It just wasn't allowed.'

'They did not let me', 'I was not allowed' . . . you would think these two phrases would be confined to the history books. And yet thirty-two years later, they were to become part of the fabric of my own first daughter's birth story, when I was 'not allowed' a home birth but instead 'had to' be induced because I was past my expected due date, and then 'had to' have a forceps delivery, because current policy 'did not let me' spend longer than two hours in the pushing stage. There were countless other small incidents during my pregnancy, labour and birth in which what was about to happen to me was presented as 'policy' or 'procedure'. The professionals I met were kind and caring, but I did not feel like I had been given a choice.

As a new mother, I contemplated all of this as I sat on my stitches and nursed my newborn in the long, isolated hours so typical of modern motherhood. I wondered – as an educated woman with a reputation for being 'opinionated', 'persistent', even 'nasty' (depending on the viewpoint of the observer) – how had this happened to me? I had laboured, as I had wanted to, free and naked, in a nest of blankets and cushions on the hospital floor. I had groaned and chanted, unfettered by drugs. I had gone to the abyss and fought my demons, as many labouring women need to do. And as I lay on that floor I had connected with my inner wild woman, with my maternal lineage, and with all the women who had been on this epic journey to meet their babies before me.

But somehow, I had been woken from this deep, almost hallucinatory trance, and moved from this place. A man had come and told me my time was up. I had been taken to the bed. I had been made to put on a shirt and cover my breasts. My feet had been placed in stirrups. I had said no to all this, but I had been told I 'must'.

At the moment of birth, I called out, in almost sexual tones, 'Oh, yes!', as my daughter's body finally slipped free. It's true, it did feel like the most perfect, ecstatic release, but the way I vocalised it was quite conscious and deliberate. It was a clear message. I wanted the doctor to know that he had not taken this pleasure from me. I had been sanitised, covered up, conventionalised, conformed: this declaration of pleasure was my final act of rebellion.

The memory of this rather strangely timed two-finger salute to my obstetrician is evidence to me, as I look back on that day just over a decade later, that even in that moment, I already knew I'd been hoodwinked. Even though I had gone into the hospital with an academic understanding of many of the feminist issues that surround modern birth, and with the desire to avoid unnecessary intervention, I had somehow ended up with my feet in stirrups. It almost felt like I had become a living metaphor: the wild woman tamed, the naked woman clothed, the renegade woman cut, the mad woman put firmly back in the attic. No wonder I made that final rebel yell.

## The Language of Permission

In the months and years that followed I began to listen to other women's birth stories with a keen ear, waiting to hear for the tipping point where they had either triumphed or, as I had, slipped beneath the waves. In every story from across the Western world I heard the same words over and over: 'They did not let me', and 'I was not allowed'. I heard it so much so that I gave this phenomenon its own special name, 'The Language of Permission'.

'I had to have a vaginal exam, as soon as I arrived at the hospital, to check if I was in labour.'

'I wanted to have a water birth, but I was not allowed to use the birth centre* because of my BMI, so I had to be on labour ward.'

'Because I was trying for a VBAC,** I was not allowed to eat or drink in labour, in case I ended up having another caesarean.'

'My partner wanted to come with me for that part, but he was not allowed.'

'They don't let you have skin to skin with your baby after a caesarean in my hospital.'

'They told me not to push yet even though I was desperate to.'

… and so it went on.

I began to wonder how these phrases were tripping so readily off our tongues as women of the twenty-first century. We would not accept being restricted in this way in our relationships or marriages, in our educational choices, or in our career paths. Why, when it came to giving birth – arguably a pretty significant moment in a woman's life – were we using such passive language, casting ourselves as the 'permission seekers', rather than the 'permission givers'?

The answer to why we have this imbalance of power, I've discovered, is complex, and emotional, but, if you put it in a big pot and simmer it for a long time, it boils down to a few interconnected essentials:

- Fear of birth is at an all-time high

---

\* In the UK, the birth centre, also known as a midwife led unit (MLU) offers a 'home from home' environment, with calm lighting and décor, birth pools, and care from midwives. If obstetric care is needed then transfer to hospital (which is sometimes located alongside the MLU) is arranged.

\** Vaginal birth after caesarean

- Confusion over the rights of the fetus can cause 'risk' to trump 'autonomy'
- And finally, we live in a patriarchy.

Let's start with the fear. In the twenty-first-century birth room, everyone – women, partners, midwives and doctors alike – is, either consciously or unconsciously, terrified of birth. This fear, which a hundred years ago may have taken the form of low-level anxiety or healthy respect, has transmogrified in recent decades into full-scale panic. Where birth was once a large stray dog that you generally expect to be friendly but approach with caution, it now seems to have evolved into a many-headed monster-hound, rumoured to be loose on the moor, with occasional sightings reported in hushed tones. Like death, birth has become something we've lost touch with, that no longer takes place in our communities and that we therefore rarely see or hear. Women go to the hospital and come back with a baby, and what happens in the intervening day or two remains a somewhat terrifying mystery. If we do see birth, it's quite likely to be a representation on TV, which, as we'll explore in Chapter 6, may be a long way from accurate.

In all areas of life, fear can make prisoners of us, and birth is no different. Our fear may shape our behaviour, our expectations, and, in turn, our actual reality. In fear, we may not prepare for birth, believing it to be 'unpredictable', or we may decline to ask questions, feeling that we are powerless. In modern maternity care, medical professionals and parents-to-be alike are often found erring on the side of caution, and this defensive behaviour can be at the expense of personal freedom. Which brings us to the overlapping concern of point two, the safety of the unborn child, another key player in the birth room power imbalance. Modern maternity care is rightly focused on birth outcomes, but a good outcome is most often measured not in terms of the woman, her feelings, her experience, and her postnatal mental health, but on the idea of the 'healthy baby' – indeed, women are frequently told that this is all that matters.

Of course, for most of us, the welfare of our baby *is* the most important aspect of the birth experience, but it's interesting how this idea that it is *all* that matters has really started to trip off the tongue in the last few decades. It has become a mantra, and hidden beneath it is a rather dark, unspoken message: women do *not* matter. In a power dynamic in which you are given the message – however subtle – that your needs and feelings are of secondary importance, it can be difficult to challenge those who are perceived to be in authority, or even to voice your discomfort. New mothers who have had what feminist Naomi Wolf calls 'ordinary bad births' – or even suffered severe trauma – are told repeatedly to 'focus on their healthy baby', as this is 'what really matters', and while this may be well-meant reassurance, to many it carries the subtext, 'Be quiet about your bad birth now please', or, worse still, 'Aren't you grateful for your baby – don't you love them?'

There is also an assumption that 'safety' and 'health' begin and end with simply having a pulse. However, as many women who have had what may look from the outside like fairly straightforward births will reiterate, feeling that you are safe can be very subjective, and being healthy is more complicated that simply looking OK on the surface. Feelings of trauma, sadness, shame, guilt, powerlessness, violation, and regret pervade the postnatal experience and reach far into the future mental and emotional well-being of women, and by default their relationships not just with themselves, but with their partners and children too. Statistics vary, but traumatic birth in the UK alone is estimated to affect nearly one in three women a year,[2] with many of those – between 4 per cent and 18 per cent – going on to develop PTSD.[3] Still others may not necessarily raise their hand to feeling full-blown trauma, but, if you ask them about their birth story, will tell you of a catalogue of missed opportunities to treat them with kindness, respect or tenderness, and sometimes atrocious treatment that they would never have felt they had the right to complain about.

During pregnancy itself, women are also reminded that the pinnacle of their birth expectations should be a healthy baby, most often at times when they show signs of having done their research and thus being keen to take an active role in the decision making. 'Birth plans' are a crucible for this phenomenon – a woman who goes so far as to outline on paper what she would like to happen to her in labour will be discouraged, at best, or even openly mocked, as we saw in November 2017 when a group of doctors caused outrage on Twitter when they joked that, 'the length of the birth plan directly correlates to the length of the caesarean incision', and that laminated birth plans were only useful if the woman had a massive haemorrhage.

# Bloody difficult women

Indeed, 'laminated' birth plans (which, in reality, I am yet to come across) seem to stand as a metaphor for a really organised and strong-minded woman who misguidedly thinks she can have any power in the birth room. In his bestselling memoir, *This is Going to Hurt*,[4] former obstetrician Adam Kay recollects a woman with a 'nine page birth plan, in full colour and laminated', who has abandoned it – 'hypnotherapy has given way to gas and air has given way to an epidural' – and is now headed for surgery due to 'failure to progress'. This, he says, does not surprise him: 'Two centuries of obstetricians have found no way of predicting the course of a labour, but a certain denomination of floaty-dressed mother seems to think she can manage it easily', is his summary.

Such attitudes pervade modern maternity care. I hear them embedded in women's birth stories daily, but if you don't believe me, you only need to look at the media reaction to celebrity births to find more of the same. My first ever paid gig as a journalist was to write about how the press were bullying Kate Middleton about her plans for a natural labour and hypnobirthing, and we've seen similar mockery of Meghan Markle in the run-up to the birth of her first baby. 'A doula and a willow tree,' a leading obstetrician apparently joked, 'let's see how that goes!'[5] The willow tree, like the floaty dress, is an attempt to poke fun at 'earth mothers' who want everything to be 'natural', and neatly portrays Meghan as demanding enough to want a particular kind of tree at her birth. It's all intended as humour, but underneath the surface is the rather chilling idea that a kind of satisfaction or sense of triumph might be gained from seeing a woman's ideal hopes for her birth go to the wall.

In Ireland, the Eighth Amendment – which gives the pregnant woman and the fetus equal rights in law – has recently been repealed, but the legacy of hundreds of years of blurred lines between Church and State mean that women's rights in birth still have a long way to go. Here, midwives in Dublin reliably inform me, a woman with a birth plan and strong ideas about what she wants is commonly referred to as 'a difficult woman' by her care team. Indeed, in early 2018 an obstetrician from a Dublin maternity unit, Dr Aoife O'Malley, described women who make birth plans as 'middle-class birthzillas', adding that her audience of fellow birth workers would 'know the women because we've all had them' who 'think they are the only woman who's ever given birth and they certainly think they are the only woman giving birth in the labour ward that day'[6].

Selfish, opinionated, controlling and difficult: women can often be treated like wayward children when they try to create this grown-up document. Lawyer and board member of Human Rights in Childbirth, Bashi Hazard, has described the birth plan as 'the closest expression of informed consent that a woman can offer her caregiver prior to commencing labour'. Hazard also reminds us that the medical institutions where we birth will always have a birth plan themselves; 'one driven purely by care providers and hospital protocols without discussion with the woman'.[7] An intelligent consideration of birth plans reveals that they are a fantastic opportunity for women to consider their many birth options and open a meaningful dialogue with their care providers about their choices. Why would anyone find this problematic? one wonders.

There is even controversy about the label 'birth plan' itself, with some birth professionals arguing that they shouldn't be called 'plans' at all, because this gives them too rigid a feel in a situation where it is important always to be flexible. 'Women need to go with the flow in labour', we are often told, as if we have the mindset of 5-year-olds. 'Preferences' is the most oft-suggested alternative, but it's interesting to consider why the word 'plan' is the source of such anxiety, in a world where women can make plans in other areas of their lives and be considered perfectly capable of adaptability, contingency or, indeed, dealing with the emotional fallout of disappointment itself. Why must we present our needs and wishes in childbirth in the style of Oliver Twist, holding out our empty bowl tentatively and apologetically, when in fact we have the legal and moral entitlement to take the lead in every single one of our childbirth choices? Imagine if business people or our politicians spoke about their 'short- and long-term preferences' – we would quickly lose confidence in their strength and leadership. Indeed, the very hospitals we give birth in have 'policies' and 'protocols', and nobody is asking them to tone that language down.

Regardless of what a woman decides to call her birth plan, she can expect to receive subtle discouragement at every turn, because birth is 'unpredictable', and you 'can't really plan for it anyway'. She will be urged to 'go with the flow', rather than try to 'control' what happens to her in labour: but whose 'flow'? As midwife and academic Dr Elizabeth Newnham puts it, 'Going with the flow is fine, as long as it's the physiological flow, not the institutional flow.'[8] Debby Gould and Melissa Bruijn, founders of the Australian birth trauma organisation BirthTalk agree: 'Most women's interpretation of "going with the flow" is "to put ourselves in the hands of our health carers, and accept the interventions they suggest as inevitable, unquestionable and in our best interests". Every week we talk with women whose birth plan was to "go with the flow". And now they are contacting us for support after a traumatic birth.'[9]

Encouragement to take a passive role in birth is everywhere, but if a woman does push ahead and make a birth plan she may find the cultural prediction that it's 'pointless' coming true: in a 2016 survey from Positive Birth Movement and Channel Mum, nearly 75 per cent of respondents said that they made a birth plan, but only half of this group said that their birth plan was read by professionals, and 42 per cent said that their plan was not adhered to.[10] In some cases, plans simply have to change: you cannot have a home water birth if you develop placenta praevia, for example, but women understand these situations and when they complain about their birth plans being disregarded, this is not the kind of example they are giving. Rather, they talk about plans not being read due to a hospital shift change or because they are 'too long', or aspects of their plan which could have held in almost any situation, such as optimal clamping, minimal talking in their birth space, or keeping their placenta, not being observed, or being told at the last minute that what they are requesting is not possible, or even not allowed.

# MAKING A BIRTH PLAN LIKE A FEMINIST

### There is a point in making a birth plan

Don't let anyone tell you otherwise. There are also ways that you can approach making that plan that will make it a valid and useful document. Firstly, know that you matter. What you want matters. You are important and your needs are important. This is your body, and your birth.

### Knowledge is power

The process of making a plan will in itself educate you on your options and get you thinking about what YOU want – that's a reason to make one right there.

### Shoot for the moon but also consider the stars

Just as you plan to party on the beach but know where the nearest cafe is if it rains, you should also think about birth plans in this way. Make a Plan A that sums up your hopes for your ideal birth. Don't be afraid to have a strong vision of what you want – with birth, as with all other areas of your life, a strong vision can help you reach your goal – but it's not a guarantee. So, once you've got that vision, make contingency plans – a Plan B (and maybe a C or D). Think about what you might want if birth deviates in any way from Plan A. Consider as many eventualities as you can.

## Ask for what you want even if it is not what others want

Only one person can have this baby, and that's you. Because of this, you absolutely get to call the shots on how and where you want it to happen. This is about you, and what you need. If you think your mum being in the room will make you feel loved and safe, great. If you think it will make you feel self-conscious and anxious – she's barred. If you want a certain type of birth – be that a home birth or a caesarean – but family members don't agree, show them the evidence behind your choice, and stick to your guns. It's your party.

## A birth plan is not 'all or nothing'

There are some parts of a plan that should only go out the window in exceptional circumstances. For example, if you want skin-to-skin contact immediately after your baby is born, or optimal clamping, this should be available in almost every circumstance. Make sure you are clear with your partner and your care providers that, even if your birth veers a long way off track, there are still some choices that you want to be honoured, no matter what.

## Make a full plan for caesarean, whether you hope to have one or not

There are lots of choices that you can make if your birth takes place in the operating theatre. Learn about 'woman-centred caesarean' and think about what might be important to you in a surgical birth. Then make a full caesarean plan.

## Make a postnatal plan

Think about what you want the first hour after birth to be like and lay out what is important to you in that time as part of your plan. You may also like to make a separate postnatal plan too, with a clear idea of how you are going to navigate the first few weeks with your baby, and a list of useful numbers for help and support with feeding.

## Get it read, get it signed!

Make sure that everyone involved in your birth reads your birth plan in advance of your labour. Your partner, doula, and any other birth supporters need to have a clear idea of what you want on the day. Discuss your plan in advance with health care providers especially if you have specific needs or requests that deviate from the norm. Ask them to record details of conversations and decisions you have made in your notes and to sign your birth plan. These discussions will help your care providers to demonstrate that they have fulfilled their obligation to have a balanced and individual discussion with you about your personal circumstances and risk factors, and you can demonstrate that you have understood the information given to you and that your wishes have been documented. Your birth plan will not have legal status, but it is still evidence that your views and preferences have been discussed and noted.

In the worst of cases, birth plans – and the questions to care providers that usually accompany them – can be interpreted as a sign of lack of care or ill will towards the unborn child, of being a 'bad mother', because of course, as a woman is repeatedly told, what happens in the birth is unimportant, as long as there is a healthy baby at the end of it. 'I wanted to know more about why they wanted to induce me, but in the end the doctor just said, "You've waited a long time for this baby, haven't you?" ', Laura from the UK told me. 'He was questioning my desire to be a mother, he was questioning how much I cared about my baby, and even how much I wanted them to live. It was a horrible moment but at that point I decided to comply with the hospital's wishes.'

Some birth workers refer to this practice as 'playing the dead baby card',[11] and it is certainly a dimension of the current fear-based climate that can be very effective in silencing a woman who is trying to argue her right to make her own choices about her body. Michelle Quashie, a mum of four from London, recalls her obstetrician similarly 'shroud waving' when she was determined to have her third baby via VBAC: 'He asked me, in quite a dramatic tone, "What is more important to you, a natural birth, or being a mother to your other children?" and as he did so he looked very pointedly at my husband as if to say, "take charge of her".' Michelle's story is reminiscent of the remarks of Irish obstetrician Dr Donal O'Sullivan who caused controversy when he said during a radio interview in 1996 that, if a woman wanted a home birth, her husband ought to put a harness on her and drive her to hospital like cattle.[12]

*A part of me, even then, could not tolerate passivity,*
*but I identified that part with the 'unwomanly' and in*
*becoming a mother I was trying to affirm myself as a*
*'womanly woman'. If passivity was required, I would*
*conform myself to the expectation.*

Adrienne Rich, *Of Woman Born*[13]

Telling women not to try to plan birth but instead to focus on the end result carries the underlying message that a woman in labour must ultimately sacrifice herself – her hopes, needs, desires, dignity or even her life – in order to save her baby. This is interesting, because, although you might assume most women would happily give their lives for their unborn if they had to, this is not always the case. If you ask pregnant women – and their partners – this rather unpleasant question, 'You can only save one, who do you save?' they will almost overwhelmingly tell you, 'the woman'. And yet, for historical, moral and religious reasons that we will explore later in this book, maternity care can often be clouded by the notion that the safety of the baby always takes precedence.

## Safety first?

In some notable cases, we can gain a window (albeit one we would rather not have) into what happens when total priority is given to the life of the baby over the wishes of the mother. In April 2014 I was privileged to speak[14] – via an interpreter – to Adelir Carmen Lemos de Góes, a 29-year-old Brazilian woman who, when expecting her third baby after two caesareans, had researched VBAC and become interested in giving birth naturally, with the help of a doula. In early labour, she attended the hospital for a check-up only to be told that her baby was in the breech (bottom down rather than head down) position. Doctors demanded she stay and have her baby by caesarean, but she signed papers to discharge herself, and left, saying she would return when her contractions were five minutes apart.

Later that night, her labour intensifying, she was picking out a dress to wear to the hospital when she saw headlights outside the windows of her house. After overhearing incredulous expressions from her husband and doula, she told me, she decided to go outside herself. 'There I was confronted by a justice officer, who stood up in front of me and said that I had to be transported to the hospital mandated by a court order that he had in his hands.'

Doctors had that afternoon obtained a court order for a compulsory caesarean.

'The whole discussion was so surreal, everything was so unbelievable and we were just trying to understand. There were about nine policemen and they were all trying to make my husband get back . . . and just take me away.' Adelir, by now experiencing strong contractions, agreed to go with them: 'I couldn't refuse – it was either do what the court order said or be handcuffed. And I was so scared – frightened with my whole body . . . having chills in my whole body.'

Adelir was driven to the nearest hospital and, although she was 9 cm dilated and nearly ready to push, her baby was born by caesarean as the court order dictated. Her husband was not allowed to be with her and she did not see him until six hours later. 'Everything had happened so suddenly and I felt pretty much robbed and kidnapped,' she told me.

Adelir's story is extreme, made more shocking, perhaps, by the fact that there was no question over her 'capacity' – she was felt to be of sound mind, but simply judged to be 'wrong' in her decision to try to birth naturally. Interestingly, when I discussed Adelir's story at the time with others, two questions repeatedly arose: 'What were the risks of the VBAC then?' and, 'How about this breech thing, didn't that make it more dangerous?' Questions like this miss the point: by trying to judge the rightness or wrongness of her decision, we fall into the same trap as the Brazilian authorities – declaring that a grey zone exists in which a pregnant woman can be compelled to make the decision that others judge is best for her, regardless of what she would choose for herself. As human rights barrister and founder of UK charity Birthrights Elizabeth Prochaska put it to me at the time of Adelir's story:

'Risk might sound appealingly scientific and rational, but it is not. When it is used to compel women to receive medical interventions, it is an expression of violent patriarchy, pure and simple. Would a Brazilian court order a man to undergo an invasive kidney transplant to save his dying child? No. Only women's bodies are treated as public objects subject to the whims of the medical profession backed by the coercive power of the state.'

Some may feel that a pregnant woman should not have the right to make a decision that puts her baby 'at risk', but, unfortunately, as unpleasant as it may sound, the unborn child can never and should never be considered to have any rights – and as soon as we put so much as a toe in this water, we begin to stray into a place in which a woman can be taken from her house by the police and compelled to undergo major surgery against her wishes. There is a creeping nature to such a mindset – once we begin to make provision for the occasions when doctors or the state may overrule a pregnant woman with full mental capacity, we are on a very slippery slope indeed. Instead, the point needs to be made clear, often over and over again, that we have to trust women to be the ultimate decision maker in birth, no matter what. This is enshrined in law, and in global principles of human rights, that I will outline in more detail in Chapter 7.

For now, let me simply share the words of the UK Court of Appeal in a case known as MB, in 1997, which could not put it more clearly:

'A competent woman, who has the capacity to decide, may, for religious reasons, other reasons, for rational or irrational reasons or for no reason at all, choose not to have medical intervention, even though the consequence may be the death or serious handicap of the child she bears, or her own death.'[15]

That sounds pretty definitive – and yet more than twenty years on, women are still asking 'Am I allowed?' in their birth space. The reason this power imbalance continues to pervade, and indeed the roots of everything this chapter has already laid out, can be found in the fact that we live in a patriarchy.* With the hashtag #metoo snowballing on social media in late 2017, a sudden uprising of women has collectively been saying, 'Keep your hands off us from now on, unless WE say so.' A vital and public conversation has been started about women's bodily autonomy, consent, and the power imbalance and patriarchal structures that, for too long, have been enabling men to behave in ways that make women feel everything on the spectrum between mildly uncomfortable and downright violated. We now need to turn the #metoo spotlight on the experience of childbirth.

## #metoo: the power of No

Currently we are only just beginning to acknowledge that we have a big, ongoing problem with the way we treat women in our culture, with our collective relationship to their bodies, with our respect for their bodily autonomy, and with consent. We would be foolish to think that women's experience of maternity care is somehow exempt from this.

Let's look at vaginal exams (known as VEs). During labour, at regular intervals – usually around every four hours – a midwife or doctor will place fingers inside you and estimate the dilation of your cervix. In this way, the speed with which your body is opening up to allow your baby to be born can be neatly marked on a graph

---

\*     Patriarchy – a society built and run by men with men's needs uppermost – affects the structures, behaviours and thoughts of everyone living within it, male and female. Even in a female-dominated profession such as midwifery, the influence of the patriarchy will be powerful and pervasive.

and your progress – or lack of it – can be readily assessed. You may be asked to lie on your back to have the VE, or get out of the birth pool. If there is any kind of 'hold up' with your labour, a VE can be a very helpful assessment, but standard practice is to perform VEs routinely, even if labour is patently 'cracking on' and there are no concerns for either woman or baby. Some women don't mind them, some really like knowing their dilation, others find them intrusive, distracting, uncomfortable, or violating. No matter how you feel about them, they are part of a standard package, and you will get them anyway.

The interesting thing about VEs is that they are completely optional – but not a lot of people know this. You would think it would be obvious – of course nobody can put their fingers inside your vagina if you don't want them to, right? But the majority of women are unaware that they are perfectly entitled to decline. Furthermore, some women report a nagging sense that they *are* entitled to decline, but are unable to voice their refusal, whereas others do manage to decline but are then either directly or indirectly coerced, for example by being told they cannot be admitted to the ward or use the birth pool unless they comply, or by simply being told they 'have to' – which is of course incorrect, as you don't 'have to' allow anything to happen to your body against your wishes. Still others consent to the VE but are told afterwards that the midwife or doctor gave them a 'sweep' or broke their waters 'while they were in there'. Women to whom this happens report finding it extremely violating and yet rarely complain formally about it, perhaps because there is a widespread and unspoken acceptance that maternity care requires you to 'leave your dignity at the door' and can at times be violating by its very nature.

Of course, you may actively *want* a VE, or indeed any other birth intervention. Giving birth like a feminist isn't about declining everything, it's about knowing that you can, and the shift in the power dynamic this brings. To use another example, in your sexual relationship, you hopefully know that if you say no to your partner at any point, they will respect your wishes. You may have been with your partner for just a few years, or for decades, and in all that time you might never have said no to them, not once. You might have said yes, yes, YES to everything! But all along, you have known that, if you wanted to say no, you could say it, and be respected. Just think how the power balance of your relationship would change if this fundamental and often unspoken understanding was not in place? And yet this is the exact dynamic in which the majority of Western women give birth.

## Good girls

There is a wider issue of compliance to those in 'white coats' that can affect all of us and is not purely a women's issue. Most of us, male and female, have been conditioned to accept without question that 'doctor knows best' and to follow their 'orders'. However, there is something about being female that makes challenging authority of any kind particularly difficult, perhaps because, as young girls looking around us as we grow, most of 'authority' *is* male. Politicians, lawyers, scientists, doctors, artists, philosophers: the default human-on-a-plinth is almost always male, and we grow up looking up to them and, consciously or unconsciously, absorbing maleness as synonymous with 'leader'. The feminist campaigner Caroline Criado Perez has tackled this head-on, getting the first statue of a woman – Millicent Fawcett – in Parliament Square, along with Jane Austen commemorated on the new £10 note, but even in the twenty-first century, these are notable exceptions – and it's worth remembering too that Criado Perez has been vilified in the media[16] and even sent death threats for her activism in this area.

As women, the social conditioning of a world dominated by men comes in tandem with consistent messages that compliance makes us more favourable humans. From birth, or even before, our culture encourages us to give girls toys, books and movies that suggest that being a girl has some connection to being passive rather than active, and conformist rather than confrontational. Even if we try to escape this as parents, our daughters will inevitably be given 'home and beauty' based toys of mirrors, cleaning equipment and plastic food, and often taught to sit neatly with their legs together, quite literally taking up less space than their male counterparts. Shoes, bags and even duvet sets are targeted at specific genders and carry similar messages: the emblem of the girl is the shy and gentle butterfly, while boys have dinosaurs and sharks as their totem animals. Even the clothes we are socially encouraged to choose for our daughters, and that they in turn are encouraged to choose for themselves, hold them back – and I speak as a mother who has spent many hours in parks watching little girls struggle to navigate climbing frames in a dress, while the boys are already ahead in their more practical and durable fabrics. Perhaps due to this early conditioning, once they hit school age girls are generally better at 'self-control' than boys,[17] and hence will be praised more consistently for being 'good', which tends to mean, 'quiet', 'still' and 'not challenging'.[18]

Believe it or not, although you may not have been referred to as a 'good girl' for at least a couple of decades, you may well find the phrase returning to your life if you are pregnant, and even – yes, really – you may hear it loud and clear while you are 'pushing' your baby out. In February 2018 medical student Natalie Mobbs, NICE fellow Catherine Williams, and Professor of Maternal Health at the University of Liverpool Andrew Weeks – wrote an opinion piece for the *British Medical Journal* entitled 'Humanising Birth',[19] about the use of language in maternity care. In it they called on health professionals to consider more carefully the words they used to pregnant and labouring women, and alongside several other problematic examples, they called out the phrase 'good girl' as disrespectful to women as autonomous adults.

'While some may mourn the days when the doctor was in charge and their advice was gratefully received and unchallenged, there are now multiple, alternative sources of healthcare advice available to women both before and after consultations. With improved knowledge among women and a renewed recognition of respect for human rights in childbirth, comes an equalisation of status between doctor and woman,' they wrote, concluding, 'The role of birth attendant is no longer "owner" of the situation but "facilitator" of the health services.'

# LANGUAGE OF MATERNITY CARE TO CALL OUT OR CHALLENGE

| Language Used | Why it's wrong | Alternatives |
|---|---|---|
| Delivered | Pizzas are delivered, babies are born. And if they are delivered, it's the woman who delivers them, nobody else! | Gave birth<br><br>Caught e.g. 'Dad caught the baby' |
| Am I allowed?<br><br>They did not let me | Women have the moral and legal right to make decisions about their birth. They cannot be compelled to make certain choices, nor should they have options denied to them. If anyone does any 'allowing', it's the woman. | I am allowed |
| Failure to progress | Nobody 'fails' at birth | Slow labour |
| Only three centimetres | Using negative language to describe the progress of labour can make some women feel discouraged, at a time when they need to be positive. | Three centimetres already, that's great! |
| My induction in room 3 | Reducing women to the intervention they are experiencing or the type of birth, etc. dehumanises them. Saying 'my' implies possession. | Say her name |

| Trial of scar | Used to describe a VBAC. Will there be a judge in a wig? | VBAC or just 'birth' |
| --- | --- | --- |
| Good girl | It's infantilising. Is this Saint Trinians? | Fantastic, that's really helpful, thanks |
| I consented her | Consent is actively given by the woman, not obtained while she remains passive. | She gave her consent |
| I just need to get your consent | Decisions should be made by the woman after full information is given and she should be made aware that she can decline or consent. | These are your choices ... the benefits and risks are ... would you like more information before you decide what you wish to do? |
| I'm just going to ... | This assumes consent has been given | I would recommend that we do x,y,z. The alternatives are ... etc. |
| She says Mum says | The woman is an individual with a name. | Use her name |

Although Mobbs, Williams and Weeks challenged a range of phrases, the UK tabloid press, who, as you can imagine, didn't like one bit the thought that infantilising and patronising women was off the menu, seized upon 'good girl' with a series of headlines in which the use of shouty capitals expressed their outrage. They even reported that midwives were now 'BANNED'[20] from using the phrase – which is not true, of course – the *BMJ* article was merely an opinion piece. It's interesting to ponder the roots of this outrage, and whether they wind their way down deep to what seems to be a cultural vested interest in the existing power imbalance; an underlying need for women in the birth room to continue to be, like the little children on the schoolroom mat, 'quiet', 'still' and 'not challenging'. Does birth as we know it rely on our silence and complicity to function, just – as we have seen from #metoo – as the wider world often does?

Being called a 'good girl' makes women feel everything from uncomfortable to outraged,[21] and while it may seem like a trivial detail to some, it is representative of paternalistic attitudes that pervade maternity care and come from care-givers of both genders. It reflects a desire to assert power over the birthing woman, who, in order to meet the expectations of her attendants and therefore show herself to be a 'good girl', must remain childlike, behave herself and comply. Often, it is when the woman tries to break free of this dynamic and take the role of 'permission giver' rather than 'permission seeker', that we see a similar kind of outrage to that expressed in the tabloid 'good girl' headlines being played out in the birth room itself.

'I went in with a suspected hind-water leak and the doctor examined me and told me they would give me steroids and antibiotics and admit me overnight,' Maryellen Stephens told me. 'I said no, that I would rather have an ultrasound, I was calm but assertive. She immediately began telling me that my baby would die and quoting a study, which I happened to have read myself. When I suggested that the study only involved ten women and wasn't really good enough evidence to extrapolate to every single birthing woman, she was enraged, and – literally – stamped her foot and stormed out. She returned with the head obstetrician who was much more measured, agreeing to my plan of coming back in the morning for an ultrasound.' Another mother, Hayley, told me her obstetrician said she was 'washing her hands of her', because she wanted to wait to be induced until the next morning. Similarly, Emily, from Southampton, told a tale I've heard multiple times: 'I was told there were not enough midwives available for my home birth, but I refused to go to hospital, knowing that I had a right to have my baby where I wished. When they finally sent two midwives, they consistently tried to find reasons to transfer me and told me my baby might die if I didn't. I stayed put and everything was fine but it really affected my experience negatively.'

Professional childbirth attendants, known as doulas, present as a supporter to the mother in the birth room and observing rather than taking any kind of active role, often report this phenomenon of women being admonished when they try to assert themselves. Interestingly, they also report how they themselves are silenced when they try to support women's autonomy. 'I have witnessed doctors becoming everything from irritated to enraged when a woman "talks back" about her options,' one UK doula told me. 'And if a doula expresses a view or backs up her client she will often be told, "I wasn't talking to you, I was talking to my patient," or worse, threatened with being reported or removed from the birth room.' Another confirmed: 'On one occasion I was told, "Don't talk for the patient" as the doctor put on their gloves and went ahead with a vaginal exam my client had not consented to. Another time I quoted the NICE guidelines and the doctor snapped, "Well clearly you know my job better than I do.'" Doulas are often gently – and sometimes harshly – mocked in the same way that birth plans are. In some countries, such as Guatemala, doulas have even been banned from the birth room, just as a notice in a Dublin hospital waiting area apparently proclaims 'You Do Not Need a Birth Plan!' Could it be that doulas, just like birth plans, speak up for the mother and her rights in a way that threatens the status quo?

# Obstetric violence

'Shut up, close your mouth and push: there is only one voice in this room, and it is mine',[22] a doctor told a mother in Illinois in 2008, and, in 2013, his words were echoed in a California birth room when a young woman named Kimberly Turbin[23] gave birth to her first child. Like many twenty-first-century labours, a home movie was made by a family member. A two-time rape survivor, Kimberly had urged her care providers to treat her gently and to explain to her every detail of what was happening. As her baby began to crown, her doctor, who had been sitting on a stool between her legs, announced he was going to perform an episiotomy (a cut to enlarge the vaginal opening). Pleading with him that she wanted more time to push her baby out naturally, Kimberly repeatedly said no. The situation in the birth room became more heated as both the doctor, the nurse, and Kimberly's own mother all urged her to comply.

On the movie, which has since been viewed over half a million times, Kimberly can be heard begging, 'No! Why? Why can't we try?'

as the doctor's voice becomes more aggressive, telling her, 'Listen: I am the expert here,' and mocking her suggestion that she can do it herself, telling her, 'You can go home and do it. You go to Kentucky.' Just to clarify, Kimberly was not from Kentucky – he meant it as a slur and an implication of 'backwardness'.

The doctor then proceeds to perform the episiotomy with twelve audible cuts to her perineum.

It's harrowing viewing. Perhaps more harrowing is the thought that Kimberly is very much not alone: a survey in 2013 by Childbirth Connection[24] found that 6 out of 10 US episiotomies were performed without consent. What makes Kimberly's case unusual is not that her body was violated in the name of expertise and safety, but that a) she had this violation entirely captured on camera and that b) she was determined to fight back. With the help of advocacy organisation Improving Birth, Kimberly went in search of a lawyer to take her case. It's notable that this in itself took 18 months. 'It took us a year and a half to find a lawyer, in spite of clear, video evidence of blatant disregard and abuse,' Dawn Thompson of Improving Birth explained. 'This should be really concerning for a lot of people! Women are coming to us and talking about coercion, manipulation, abuse – every single day, and some of it is just being accepted because it's just considered par for the course of giving birth in our current maternity care system.'

'Many of the lawyers we've spoken to are not sure whether a woman giving birth has the right to say "No" to a medical procedure,' her colleague Cristen Pascucci told me during their search for legal representation. 'And they don't see the dollar value in litigating this kind of a case, when they know that, just like them, any jury probably believes that the best outcome of childbirth is a live baby – irrespective of whether the mother has been maimed by her care providers in the process.'

Eventually the case was settled out of court in 2017, amidst wide praise for Kimberly for highlighting the issue of consent and abuse in the birth room. Her attorney, the prominent civil rights lawyer Mark Merrin, called the lawsuit, 'a big step for women who have been silenced'. It's easy to see this story as an isolated case, or to conceptualise it as an American problem, but, unfortunately, it's just one example of a widespread, global issue, referred to as 'obstetric violence'.

It's worth saying at this point that the term 'obstetric violence', perhaps understandably, tends to push buttons and cause misunderstanding, first and foremost because people mistakenly think that 'obstetric' implies it is only perpetrated by obstetricians. In fact, 'obstetric' simply means 'relating to childbirth and the processes associated with it', and the term therefore covers any violation a woman experiences in the birth setting. The second word in the term – 'violence' – also causes confusion. While people are generally able to accept that pushing or hitting or maliciously hurting a person is 'violence', when a professional is 'just doing their job' and 'helping the baby to be born safely', for example by insisting they stay on the bed when they really want to move, it is harder to understand this as a violent act. Nor do we always understand acts of coercion, emotional or psychological abuse, lack of proper consent, misuse of power, or abusive or unkind language as acts of 'violence'. Indeed, as we have seen in the case of Kimberly Turbin, even when the act is quite clearly aggressive and violent towards the woman, there is a kind of cultural blind spot that allows us, for the most part, to accept it as 'just what birth is like'.

Kimberly's case is an extreme example of obstetric violence; there are also many other more subtle ways in which a woman can feel violated during her birth experience, and they are all equally valid. It might be helpful for everyone if obstetric violence were instead called 'obstetric abuse' or even 'birth abuse', in order for everyone to understand fully just what and who is encompassed by this broad term. However, too much debate around the semantics can evolve into a distraction from the solid fact: this is happening to women, and we need to hear their voices. Perhaps, as Mila Oshin, the director of the Digital Institute for Early Parenthood (DIEP), put it at a Birth Trauma conference I attended in 2018, we need to accept that those who have not experienced obstetric violence are last on the list to decide how it should be named. 'The term obstetric violence is one that does not necessarily reflect the intentions of others, but I feel entitled to use it in reference to my experience,' she said.

Thanks to Latin American birth activists, Venezuela is the first country formally to define obstetric violence, making it one of nineteen kinds of punishable violence against women. It's helpful to read their definition and consider how it applies to our own experiences of maternity care, wherever we may be in the world.

*The appropriation of a woman's body and reproductive processes by health personnel, in the form of dehumanizing treatment, abusive medicalization and pathologization of natural processes, involving a woman's loss of autonomy and of the capacity to freely make her own decisions about her body and sexuality, which has negative consequences for a woman's quality of life.*[25]

The following list, from Venezuelan law, of what constitutes obstetric violence, is also helpful. They state that it encompasses:

- untimely and ineffective attention to obstetric emergencies
- forcing the woman to give birth in a supine position when the necessary means to perform a vertical delivery are available
- impeding early attachment of the child with his/her mother without a medical cause
- altering the natural process of low-risk labour and birth by using augmentation techniques
- performing caesarean sections when natural childbirth is possible, without obtaining the voluntary, expressed, and informed consent of the woman.[26]

Both action and inaction can be violent, and violating. Neglecting a woman in labour who is asking for pain relief or stating that something is wrong, denying access to a caesarean, or intervening too late,[27] could be considered acts of violence, just as the 'too much too soon'[28] approach can also be violent, undermining a woman's autonomy and depriving her of the chance to experience her own bodily capabilities. The World Health Organisation (WHO) has also called for the prevention and elimination of abuse and disrespect during childbirth, and the reduction of unnecessary intervention, stating that, 'The growing knowledge on how to initiate, accelerate, terminate, regulate, or monitor the physiological process of labour and childbirth has led to an increasing medicalisation of the process. It is now being understood that this approach may undermine a woman's own capability in giving birth and could negatively impact her experience of what should normally be a positive, life-changing experience.'[29] As Dr Princess Nothemba Simelela, WHO Assistant Director-General for Family, Women, Children and Adolescents, put it in February 2018, 'A "good birth" goes beyond having a healthy baby.'[30]

Women who say they have experienced obstetric violence normally describe situations where they feel their personhood has been disregarded, their voice has not been heard, they have not been properly informed of what is happening to them, they have not given their consent to a procedure, or they feel that their body boundaries have been transgressed without permission. They often use the language of rape and violation, reflecting the sexual and intimate nature of the birth process. In many cases they feel they have been treated with straightforward cruelty or disrespect, but at times they also express an understanding that the professionals in charge of their care were 'doing what they had to do', but that they could have done this in a way that made them feel more involved, informed, and respected: 'This would not have taken much time but it would have made all the difference to me.' Often, the health professionals' superior knowledge is used as a justification for proceeding against the woman's wishes: as one doctor told his patient, 'I have delivered hundreds of babies, you have not delivered any'.[31]

It's very important to be clear that the vast majority of medical staff do not knowingly perpetrate obstetric violence. This is because, as academics and experts in obstetric violence Sara Cohen Shabot[32] and Keshet Korem point out, obstetric violence is 'structural' not 'behavioural': 'the staff merely perpetuate the violence of the existing structure'.[33] In other words, this way of behaving towards labouring women is not only institutionalised but also held up and perpetuated by our culture, and, like other gender-based violence and abuse, accepted as normal and allowed to go unchallenged. Health care workers will almost certainly not be aware of how their behaviours towards women are experienced, unless we find our voices and tell them. We also need to challenge the 'small' attitudes and actions that underpin obstetric violence. 'Locker room banter' is not rape, but it does normalise misogyny and, by extension, violence against women. Likewise jokes that mock or degrade labouring women help to prop up a system in which disrespect and abuse take place, and we should therefore continue to challenge them just as we challenge all other 'everyday sexism'. Every single denial of a woman's autonomy and power in the birth room, great or small, is part of the same problem. Call it out.

Interestingly, and also in common with other forms of violence against women, it is often the woman who is left carrying the blame and shame in the aftermath. Just as the woman who has been attacked may feel that the clothes she wore or the route she took home at the end of the night may have contributed to her violation, women traumatised by birth will spend the days, weeks or even years afterwards going over the events in fine detail and asking, 'What could I have done differently?' And, just as men are rarely asked to reflect on what they could do to reduce violence against women there is similarly considerably less postnatal analysis – and often none at all – done by the individuals, institutions and systems that inflict birth trauma. Women are left with the shameful reflection that they 'should not have got their hopes up', 'should not have made a birth plan', or 'should have just gone with the flow' and these messages are consistently reinforced in popular culture. Those who try to take control of their births, and antenatal courses and teachers who encourage them to believe they can do so, are consistently derided and mocked. 'Yes,' the woman thinks to herself, 'I was totally unrealistic to think I could have a positive experience of birth, and that is why I now feel so awful. It is *my* fault I feel this way.' This is victim-blaming, pure and simple.

## 'Can I hold her now?' Who owns the baby?

In 2018 research into skin-to-skin contact after caesarean, academics observed the mother's body was perceived to be divided after the birth, with obstetricians 'owning' the bottom half, anaesthetists 'owning' the top half, and midwives 'owning' the baby.[34] Mothers may wish to hold their newborns desperately, but in both caesarean and vaginal births, the first hands to touch the baby are often not the woman who birthed them, and she may have to wait to hold them. Often, in a vaginal birth, the moments directly before the birth will have been strictly controlled by the professionals, too, with the woman being told when and how to push, or even instructed not to push at all until given permission. And the imbalanced power dynamic does not end with the arrival of the baby. One question I have been asked many times by pregnant women is 'What do I do if I want to keep my placenta? Am I allowed?' It's fascinating to me that women are uncertain about this, when clearly the placenta belongs to them and came from their own body, just like the baby. This permission-seeking speaks volumes about the dynamics of power in birth and about the background against which we see the violation of women and their bodies being normalised on a daily basis. Just as the baby was once whisked off to the hospital nursery without so much as a by your leave, the placenta (in many cultures considered a meaningful or even sacred organ) is often disposed of without question or consent. Most women aren't bothered by this but that isn't really the point – the point is that, among those who *are* bothered, there is an uncertainty about ownership, and, on occasion, a violation of their rights to keep the placenta or at least be consulted about their wishes.

Similarly, the cutting of the umbilical cord has become almost symbolic of power and ownership in the birth room. Midwife Amanda Burleigh has campaigned for fifteen years for 'optimal cord clamping', sometimes called 'delayed cord clamping'.

'We know that there is plenty of evidence to support the health benefits of delayed clamping and it has been a NICE guideline since 2014,' she told me. 'However, in spite of myself and a number of others campaigning for clinicians to wait just a few minutes, some are still cutting the cord immediately which is not recommended and research shows can cause harm.'

Indeed, in a survey by the Positive Birth Movement[35] of parents whose babies were born in the UK between 2015 and 2017, nearly a third stated that their baby's cord was cut less than a minute after the birth, with one in five stating the cord was cut immediately. Arguably, cutting the cord too early with no clinical reason could be described as an act of obstetric violence, and yet it clearly continues to happen in UK birth rooms and globally – why? Some say it's just because change takes a while and 'that's the way it's always been done', others suggest that in a time-pressed world, it can be difficult to pause. I wonder. Could it be there is something about the moment of birth that is so powerful, that somehow there is an unconscious need to lay claim to the cutting of the cord and holding of the baby (perhaps the ultimate 'prize')? It is certainly very interesting to look at the behaviour of birth attendants in the first hour of life, and notice just how much disturbance can take place to the mother–baby bond and interaction.

> *It seems as if the moment the baby arrives the focus on the mother is lost. It becomes about the staff's interactions with the baby. The doctor who insisted on delivering my baby cut the cord, announced the gender and held her aloft like a hunting trophy. She illustrated her take on who was relevant in the room and who wasn't. My husband and I did not feature, let alone the baby.*
>
> Hannah Carter, UK

> *A poignant ventouse delivery – it's a mum I saw in infertility clinic at the very start of this job. I feel like holding the baby aloft like Simba and blasting out my best 'Circle of Life'.*
>
> Adam Kay, *This is Going to Hurt*[36]

I have called the first hour after the birth the 'Hour of Power'. I call it this for two reasons: partly because it's a time when, ideally, a woman should be feeling pretty triumphant, and partly because it's a 'supercharged' time in which a new human begins their first experiences of the world, and a woman and family meet that human for the first time. It's magical, and, just like birth, we should be thinking about what we can put in place to make this time special and memorable for everyone involved, and what our plan B is if this doesn't work out.* Ideally, the time should be calm and undisturbed – as pioneering obstetrician Michel Odent puts it, 'don't wake the mother'.[37] During this time a complex set of hormonal and biological processes take place that affect bonding, lactation, the colonisation of the baby's skin and gut flora, and the baby's adaptation to the world of breathing, gravity and thermo-regulation, to name just a few. Of primary importance is the hormonal dance during which the mother falls in love with her newborn; if left to their own devices, this will take place with mother and baby in skin-to-skin contact, quietly meeting one another's gaze. It's very unusual to see this unique time unfold naturally without interruption, however, and not just in Western culture, but globally – where everything from a belief that colostrum is bewitched to bathing, eye drops, suctioning the nose, swaddling or ear-piercing disrupt the golden time between parent and child.

The Hour of Power is not always experienced as empowering. In the time immediately following the birth, women most often readily accept that professionals have important checks to do that must take precedence over what is often an overwhelming and even physically felt need to hold their babies. The question 'Can I hold her now?' can be heard in birth rooms globally, as the mother seeks permission to have her newborn returned to her. Odent has

---

\* For those who for whatever reason are unable to have that first hour with their baby, I do recommend 'postponing' it rather than thinking of it as 'lost' – you can have that time of quiet skin to skin and marvelling at the beauty of your baby a week, a month or even longer after the birth if necessary, and it's still an Hour of Power.

an interesting theory about why, with our early clamping, washing, wiping, weighing, and bewitched colostrum, nobody can seem to leave mothers and babies in peace. The disruption of bonding has an evolutionary advantage, he argues, creating tougher humans and better warriors: 'The greater the social need for aggression and an ability to destroy life, the more intrusive the rituals and beliefs are in the period surrounding birth.'[38] Whether or not Odent is right, it's certainly true that Westerners value 'independence' in their children, and that the link between parenting and personality is well established. In disrupting the Hour of Power, our cultural values – that efficiency and tick boxes matter more than relationships and connection – are certainly being upheld. Furthermore, if Odent is right, we're upholding the patriarchy, too, laying the foundations for a new generation of aggressors and destroyers, who will in their turn cut, clamp, separate and generally disrupt the oxytocic peace. Whichever way you look at it, Odent sums it up well when he says, 'reconsidering our attitudes during this short period of time shakes the very foundations of our cultures'.

# Love from a distance: life in the NICU

The early attachment of woman and baby is also low on the list of priorities when a baby is born prematurely. Common practice is for the baby to be taken to a special unit and placed in an incubator, with only a few pioneering neonatal units in the world doing things differently. In Uppsala, Sweden, Dr Uwe Ewald and colleagues encourage 'kangaroo care',[39] whereby the separation of the baby from their parent is kept to a minimum. His state-of-the-art unit places babies in skin-to-skin contact on the chests of their carers, out of the incubator and in bed or often in slings, with mobile monitors in the parent's pocket. However, in Dr Ewald's experience, parents will often detect issues several seconds ahead of the monitor. Ewald's work is inspired by a focus on the rights of the child not to be separated from their parents, an understanding of early infant attachment – 'Bonding is a bit more than just holding a finger,' he points out – and an empathy for the experience of both the baby and the parents and the anguish of separation they may be feeling.

Dr Ewald's way of thinking is highly unusual, however, and the majority of parents whose babies are in the NICU will be apart from them and will often feel the need to ask, 'Am I allowed?' 'At the start we didn't realise that we were actually able to touch her,' said one mother. 'Nobody told us we were allowed and we thought it was just the nurses who could. We didn't hold her either because we didn't realise we could.' 'I did not feel like she belonged to me,' said another NICU mother, while another commented, 'I felt like I was cluttering the place up because I hung out there so much.'[40]

Donna Booth, who founded the New Zealand organisation NUMB (Neonatal Unity for Mothers and Babies) after her own experience, told me of how the imbalanced power dynamic of the NICU made her feel assaulted. 'My baby was born by caesarean and I had a general anaesthetic that I did not want. This was the first assault. The second assault happened when I was in recovery and NICU staff kept sending messages insisting on having my child's name given to them to write in the notes and on the incubator – but I wanted to be the one to name this child when I recovered. The third assault was when I finally got to the NICU in a wheelchair and the nurse (probably thinking she was being welcoming and helpful) introduced me to my baby, taking the hat off the baby and telling me the hair colour and remarking on the fingers and toes. I wanted with all of my heart and soul to be the one to discover these things myself, to reclaim this time, to marvel in the gorgeousness of my perfect child; but she stole that from me. There were further assaults. Mothers like me who want to be with their babies are a challenge for the NICU. "Parents can visit any time" does not mean you can stay for twenty-four hours a day without some sort of resistance, punishment or even being positioned as somehow not right in the head.'

## 'Re-centering me as the decision maker': love and loss

Attitudes and practices like these of Donna's NICU staff are usually well meant, but often so deeply ingrained that they are beyond everyday awareness and rarely analysed or reconsidered. They are another part of our 'allowed/not allowed' birth culture. We know that, most often, health professionals have their patient's best interests, and in particular safety, uppermost in their minds. To a clinician, everybody getting out of birth alive is the greatest priority. They have been trained to view every aspect of the experience through the framework of safety and risk, and this can sometimes be the justification for the over-medicalisation of birth or even for treatment lacking in empathy or compassion: 'There simply wasn't time' It's interesting, therefore, to look at what happens to women when these safety concerns are completely removed, in that terrible scenario of baby loss.

'Attitudes to stillbirth have improved a lot in recent times,' Mel Scott, from the charity Finley's Footprints, tells me. 'Up until the past decade or so, babies who had died tended to be whisked off immediately or after just a few minutes. I still get messages from mums who lost their baby twenty years ago, who didn't see them, hold them, name them, and don't know where they are buried. And they have never forgotten, never got over it, and always regret not having that time. Although there have been some great improvements, it's still the case that most parents don't realise they have choices they can make about how they welcome their baby, or how they spend their time together, or where their baby goes.'

Natalie Lennard, whose son Evan was stillborn in 2013, had to fight for permission to give birth to him at home, even though he had a condition – Potter's Syndrome – that meant there was absolutely nothing a hospital could have done to save him.[41] Hospital protocol was to end the pregnancy via an in-utero injection and induce the birth under epidural – choosing not to do this was a highly unusual and counter-cultural choice. With the support of Virginia Howes, an independent midwife, Natalie finally got permission to birth at home, at term, a triumphant and positive experience for her in spite of her loss: 'His nose, ankles and wrists were squashed from having no fluid around him in the womb but otherwise he was my simply perfect baby. How could I have ever wanted him whisked away, cleaned and wrapped? No way, holding his bloody birthy beautiful body in my arms was the best part of all!' Natalie is passionate that it was the support she received from her midwife that made truly informed choice possible; she was 'the only character who stood alone from any party, and kept re-centring me as the decision-maker'.

Natalie goes on to say, 'I joined a group on Facebook for Potter's Syndrome and every few months a new woman joins from somewhere in the world, whose baby will have been diagnosed with exactly what Evan had, and sometimes she terminates within a couple of days because in their words, the "doctor thought it best". Those women were never even given a choice, they probably didn't think they had one. It would have been hard enough for me even with my own determination, but these women have no one to play the role of angelic devil's advocate . . . Virginia's attitude is nothing short of revolutionary, the future of all health care.'

Currently, a revolutionary attitude, and, if possible, a 'Virginia' for back-up, is required all round if you want to birth *your* baby, from *your* body, *where* you want, and *how* you want. Elective caesarean? This might require persistence: a report from the charity Birthrights in August 2018[42] highlighted that, in spite of UK NICE guidelines supporting a woman's right to choose and be supported in this option, 15 per cent of trusts have an explicitly stated policy not to offer it, while a further 47 per cent were unclear as to whether a woman requesting a surgical birth would actually get one. The reasons for elective or maternal request caesarean are complex,[43] but in many cases requesting surgery is an attempt to take control over bodily autonomy, often after a previous birth experience where this was felt to be completely lost: 'I chose an elective for both physical and psychological reasons,' the journalist Natasha Pearlman writes. 'The thought of surgery terrified me, to be honest, but not as much as giving birth naturally again.'[44] Autonomy is also a factor for women who have a history of sexual abuse: 'I chose caesarean because it felt like, in terms of my history, it would be safer, more predictable. I didn't want anything to happen, in particular involving physical touch, where I might feel out of control as I felt this would be very triggering,' Lindsay, who had elective surgery in Australia for both her babies, told me. Maternal request caesarean forces us to ask questions about why some women would rather have major surgery than experience modern childbirth, and until at least some of those questions are addressed and resolved, there should be no barriers for the small percentage of women who request a birth in theatre.

## Opting out: freebirth

Freebirth, the choice to labour and give birth without a midwife or any other health professional present, may seem as far away from elective caesarean as it's possible to get, but, in fact, as is so often the case with opposite ends of the spectrum, they have much in common. Blogger and doula Jenny Wren has described freebirth as a 'feminist statement . . . because it is the radical notion that the woman takes priority over the baby'.[45] Several studies have been carried out into women's motivation to freebirth,[46] finding that negative experiences of maternity care are a driving factor in many cases, with one study published in the journal *BMC Pregnancy and Childbirth* concluding:

> *The UK based midwifery philosophy of woman-centred care that tailors care to individual needs is not always carried out, leaving women to feel disillusioned, unsafe and opting out of any form of professionalised care for their births. Maternity services need to provide support for women who have experienced a previous traumatic birth. Midwives also need to help restore relationships with women, and co-create birth plans that enable women to be active agents in their birthing decisions even if they challenge normative practices. The fact that women choose to freebirth in order to create a calm, quiet birthing space that is free from clinical interruptions and that enhances the physiology of labour, should be a key consideration.[47]*

Women's actual stories of freebirth support these findings. I share two here in their entirety because I think they speak volumes not just about the choice to freebirth – which only a tiny minority of women make – but about the imbalance of power and overall lack of true listening that this chapter is essentially about, and that a much wider group of women are coming across in their maternity experience.

The first is from Megan, who gave birth in the south of England. Both her births took place between 2009 and 2019.

*I have had two lovely home births. During my first birth I got the impression the NHS midwives that attended didn't want to be there. It was a busy night on the ward, I was asked to come into the hospital for a VE (vaginal exam), but I declined, I didn't want any VEs due to testing positive for Group B strep, and knowing they would increase the risk of infection and possibly rupture my waters prematurely which is another risk factor. I also have a fear of hospitals ever since witnessing the substandard care my sister experienced during her first birth. My informed choice was not respected and when the midwives did arrive at my home I was coerced into having an unwanted VE because they threatened that they couldn't stay unless they knew I was in established labour. My contractions were 3 minutes apart lasting 2 minutes by this point. It was quite clear to anyone watching that I was in established labour. I was 7 cm upon checking.*

*I was later told, during pushing, I had to get out of the pool for an episiotomy because baby was in distress and not moving down (he was having heart rate decelerations). They had me semi-reclined in the pool and were coaching me to do horrible chin-on-chest pushing. I asked to try one more thing first, I listened to my body, got myself into an upright squat and pushed my baby's head out on the next contraction with ease* and no tearing. The next contraction brought the rest of his body out and he was perfect, alert, and peacefully looking up at us both.

I was then pestered for the next 30 minutes to keep checking his cord to see if they could cut it yet (I wanted to 'wait for white'), and then once it was cut, it was more pestering about having the injection to bring the placenta out. Again I declined 2–3 times. I ended up having it tugged out of me by the cord. I had no idea how dangerous that was! There were great parts of my birth too, I wouldn't call the birth traumatic. But I didn't feel cared for by the midwives. I felt rushed and coerced into completing their tick list so that they could move on and get back to the hospital.

So during pregnancy two, as I reflected back on this birth I realised that the midwives being there didn't make me feel safe at all. And safety is important in birth. I wanted an independent midwife who I trusted and had got to know as I did my doula, but I couldn't afford one. So I wrote a detailed birth plan for the NHS midwives; no VEs, no temps, no BP, no questions, no talking, intermittent monitoring of baby's heart rate only. Basically I wanted the midwife to sit back and watch me birth my baby, as a safety net in case anything did go wrong.

*However, I got a phone call from the supervisor of midwives, who was gravely concerned at my request for a hands-off birth. She actually asked me if I would 'allow' the midwives to use oxygen on my baby if they were born not breathing! I could not believe this! How did a request for a hands-off birth get put into the same category as a mother who doesn't want any medical assistance to her baby should there be complications? After that phone call I was so angry. I lost all trust in the NHS midwives. I decided that I wouldn't be inviting anyone into my birth space until I knew the birth was imminent. As it turned out I had a virtually pain-free birth and no transition signs, I went from mild regular contractions to pushing contractions and my baby being born within 15 minutes with just me, my boyfriend, our three-year-old son and my doula present. She was perfect and healthy thankfully but I am still angry that I was put in that position because of such a rigid checklist system that we call midwifery care.*

The second birth story is from Kay Parsons, in Massachusetts, USA, whose babies were born between 2004 and 2014.

*I was 19 the first time I gave birth and felt like being young and unmarried really affected how I was treated. From the moment I arrived at the hospital I felt like my autonomy was stripped from me.*

*I so clearly remember the moment they told me that they thought he may be malpositioned or have his cord wrapped around his neck. I had taken some prenatal yoga classes and wanted to try different positions to give him space to turn or adjust but they 'wouldn't allow' me to. They forced me onto my back so they could monitor his heart rate.*

*There were so many people rushing in and out of the room. Every time I'd have a contraction, 10 people would run into the room and stare at my belly or at the monitors as though doing so would somehow change the outcome of his heart rate deceleration. Of course it did nothing to help him and made me feel like an animal on display in the zoo!*

*At one point I had five different people all holding sharp objects wanting to poke or prod me in some way. I couldn't catch my breath, started to cry, and asked for a moment to just centre myself and breathe and a nurse said to me, 'Oh honey, you can't cry now, you have so much more to come!'*

*In the end he was born by caesarean. The whole experience was so traumatic and brought to the surface past experiences of sexual trauma and the feeling of having no voice, no power, and no right to decide what is best for me or my baby.*

*When I got pregnant a couple of years later I knew that I would never feel safe having a baby in the hospital again. We hired midwives and had a lovely, but trying and long home birth. Five years later I had another midwife-assisted home birth.*

*I found that the midwives were all great. I really believe in midwife-assisted home births and have trained to become a midwife myself. But I've always struggled with feeling like even midwife-assisted births contain an element of fear and trying to control the outcome.*

*I've found that many home birth midwives are great at supporting women to labour autonomously, follow their intuition, and trust the birthing process. But even the best of midwives change when a woman starts pushing. They rush around and get a bit frantic and have their hands all up in her business. It's like they are ingrained to need to 'do something' perhaps out of fear, perhaps out of excitement, perhaps out of liability. But the energy of the room changes. Things get busy, and rushed. There's the clanking of instruments and busyness of preparing for the big moment. And I've found that their fear becomes palpable to me. Even in my trance of 'labourland' I feel pulled out into the mundane of their sense of responsibility for the outcome.*

*I read an article once about the holistic stages of childbirth that talks about the moment of pause before a baby fully arrives earthside. This quiet moment where the world stands still and they emerge into the world and I longed for that experience.*

*I didn't want anyone to rush the moment of emergence. I wanted to birth without the fear that comes with the anticipation of baby's final arrival. I wanted to savour that moment, in between the worlds, where my baby is not yet fully outside me and yet not completely within me either. So I planned a freebirth with my last baby. Just my husband, me, and two of my dearest friends.*

*And when she arrived, I had my moment. The whole world stood still. It was just me, her, my husband, and our hands as she made her way earthside. It was the most empowering moment of my life!*

*But perhaps I placed too many prayers on holding the slowness of that moment. She was a little slow to start breathing normally. It was like she sat in that pause with me for too long and when she started breathing, it was shallow and fast, like she couldn't quite catch her breath and arrive. We were nervous so we called the paramedics 'just in case'.*

*They arrived, and the two male paramedics were obnoxious and a bit freaked out, but this one woman paramedic was amazing. Before ever touching my baby, she knelt down beside me, looked me in the eye, and congratulated me before ever saying another word. She never judged me for birthing at home or birthing alone. She expressed nothing but support for my autonomy and my choices. She held the sacred with me, even if she didn't know it.*

*She encouraged me to bring her in and have her evaluated but at that point she was already breathing normally. When she found out she was my fourth baby she laughed and said, 'Never mind, mama. You got this!'*

*It was a moment of such deep healing. Of course all of the nightmare scenarios were running through my head, the fear of being judged, disempowered, having my magical moment taken from me again. And instead I was met with utter respect and trust in my knowing of my baby and my body. Somehow it healed, all the way back to that first experience of birth, and all the way forward to every moment of support I will offer another woman. Even in the midst of 'complications' this paramedic reminded me that we have the choice, to join mama in the sweetness and the stillness and treat her with respect, autonomy and trust.*

Every generation likes to think that they are free, and often, only the clarity of hindsight can reveal just how restricted they actually were. My mother, for example, like many women in the seventies, thought that it was the pinnacle of freedom to have her labour induced, to know what day of the week on which I would be born and make practical arrangements, and to have a kindly midwife look after her newborn while she rested. Looking back on it now, over four decades later, she can more easily see the restrictions placed on her personal freedom that were epitomised when, lost and drug-hazy, she wandered the hospital corridors looking for the baby she knew she had just birthed, but could not find anywhere.

It would be foolish to assume that 'that was then, this is now' and that there is nothing happening to women in twenty-first-century maternity care that will not, when we look back on it in another forty years, seem laughable or even barbaric. In fact, you don't necessarily need twenty–twenty hindsight – you only have to talk to women who are experiencing the current birth system to hear a myriad of restrictions, small and large, that are placed on their freedom, and a range of abuses, small and large, that are happening to them and hiding in plain sight in every maternity ward. When I listen to these stories, the same thought keeps coming back to me – birth needs a feminist revolution! But where is it? Where is feminism?

# Chapter 2

# Birth: the Land that Feminism Forgot?

*Women are driven through the health system like sheep through a dip. The disease they are being treated for is womanhood.*

Germaine Greer[1]

Pregnant for the first time in 2007, I kept getting flashes of Greer. For those who are unfamiliar, Greer Flashes* are a bit like hot flushes, but rather than being confined to the menopause they can occur at any time in a woman's life, when, just as she is completely preoccupied with an everyday oppression, Germaine's face will appear suddenly and without warning in her mind's eye and drawl

---

\*    Flashes may also come in the form of any leading feminist.

at her in a mild but firm Australian accent. For me, Greer Flashes really started to intensify during that pregnancy, although I'm sure that someone, somewhere, will confidently tell me that this was 'just hormones'.

Educated, articulate, professional and healthy, I guess I was used to feeling confident, and, for the most part, being treated like a grown-up. Once pregnant, however, I suddenly felt patronised, dictated to and pathologised in subtle ways that were hard to express, but which all seemed to come back to the same thing – I was constantly perceived as fragile although I felt extremely strong. I was suddenly discouraged from having my steak rare, offered seats on public transport,* and once, when putting up party decorations, cautioned for blowing up balloons and firmly told off for standing on a chair. My bump size and shape seemed under constant scrutiny, as were any birth choices I dared to give voice to. On one occasion I remember another woman watching me and declaring I was 'Sweet!' as I hungrily tucked into a curry in my local pub. I felt observed and judged in a way that I had never before experienced, and my feminist hackles began ever so slightly to rise.

Much of this, of course, was before I really entered into the maternity care system and started to experience the imbalanced power dynamics first hand. A few violent sweeps of my membranes, an episiotomy in stirrups, patchy attention paid to consent, and – the final push – hearing the many birth stories of traumatised friends,

---

\* I do realise that many people think it's a lovely thing that pregnant women are offered seats, but for me at that time, it felt odd and unnecessary.

and the Greer Flashes intensified. Just what *did* she have to say about childbirth, I wondered, feeling that if ever an area of women's lives needed some feminist action, surely this had to be it.

I'd first properly read Greer on a beach holiday in my twenties, during which – presumably because escapism is not so high on the agenda when you're 26 and working on your tan – I'd decided to eschew Jilly Cooper in favour of her new title, *The Whole Woman*. The book, a powerful 1999 'sequel' to the explosive 1970 bestseller *The Female Eunuch*, explores how, as Greer wryly puts it, women have become accustomed to spending their lives 'under the doctor', adding 'Much of what is done to women in the name of health has no rationale beyond control.'[2]

Turning back to my dog-eared and still slightly sandy copy of *The Whole Woman*, I read it again, through my new – and stereotypically knackered – mummy eyeballs. Birth was in there, but confined to just a handful of fascinating pages. In a few quick brushstrokes, Greer points out the obvious – that the disparity in intervention statistics around the world ought to be our first indicator that something was badly amiss. 'If it were true that episiotomy, caesarean section and hysterectomy were never performed except when genuinely necessary we would not expect to see such an enormous range of variation in the numbers of operations carried out in countries with much the same standards of living and health care,' she writes.

It was great to see at least a passing feminist reference to this 'postcode lottery', but I was seeing it in my immediate world at epidemic proportions, framed in the real stories of women I knew rather than enclosed in global statistics, and to date I've been unable to find much feminist outrage about it. In fact, this was later to prompt me to harness the power of social media via the Positive Birth Movement, so that women could connect with each other across geographical divides and share and compare both medical advice and personal experience. I first noticed the power of Facebook to address this problem when a friend, knowing I was a bit of a birth nut, contacted me to say, 'What do I do? This is my third baby, but this time they want to induce me because I'm 41.' When I posted on social media, Greer's postcode lottery point was suddenly brought to life as different women in different parts of the world, or even different parts of the country, shared the conflicting advice they'd been given on this issue. For some, induction was not even mentioned, for others, it was advised, for still others, it was presented as totally essential for safety. What was the true risk? Nobody seemed to know, but my friend was in the last category, and she took the induction.

In my own case, when planning a home birth with my third after a second, very big baby, I'd been told that the advice I'd receive was literally down to whether I saw the obstetrician on the left-hand side of the corridor, or the one on the right. On the left – which was the man I actually saw – a laid-back and friendly chap who wondered what I was doing there: 'You pushed out your last baby no problem, right? It was quick, you didn't tear? A home birth will be fine!' On the right, behind the door I never opened, an obstetrician renowned for 'not believing in vaginal birth', so much so that he 'made his wife have all theirs by caesarean'. How much of this was true and how much hospital mythology I cannot say, but it felt like a lucky escape that somehow simultaneously summed up the potluck nature of maternity care. We have to remember, too, that this lucky dip system has tangible and long-lasting impacts on women's lives, bodies, and mental health. It can mean the difference between major surgery or no surgery, empowerment or disempowerment, trauma or transformation, life or death. Why is there not more of a feminist fuss?

Greer had something to say about episiotomies, too, citing childbirth guru Sheila Kitzinger who called them 'our Western way of female genital mutilation'.[3] This was something I had first-hand experience of, and deeply wished I hadn't: since everything about my body 'bounced back' fairly well after birth apart from my sad and sorry scar, for a long time seeming to represent me in some way by being 'reluctant to heal', 'angry', and 'weeping'. Even now, ten years later, I can still feel it, like a little knot that reminds me not to forget. The really nagging question, for me and for all women who receive this cut, is – did I really need it? If I did, then fine. If not, then I'm frankly pretty cheesed off about it. Feminists should be demanding answers to these questions before another generation of women are unnecessarily scarred, but again, the issue seems to be off the feminist radar. Greer seems to side with the idea that a lot of intervention probably isn't needed, and that we express our lack of confidence in women and their bodies in the birth room, as we do pretty much everywhere else. She talks about how doctors 'believe that women's vaginas have such a dreadful tendency to split from stem to stern while doing the job they were designed for that they have to be surgically opened in advance to avoid a very nasty mess', and suggests that, 'one way to avoid the mutilation of episiotomy is to have one's belly cut open instead', adding, 'Many of these women will have opted for active birth only to be convinced by their attendants that the baby is struggling, that they are incompetent after all.' Greer's message is clear: women's bodies *are* fit for purpose, but we have a complete lack of understanding about how they function and have been conditioned to hand over our power to doctors. This we do without question: 'Women believe that their bodies are so mysterious that only a person in a white coat could unravel them, and so defective that there was never any hope of their functioning properly in the first place.' I cheered as I read Greer's message, which absolutely aligned with my personal experience and with the many other women's birth stories I'd heard since. But a few passing sentences written in a book twenty years ago seem to have made little impression on women's real experiences. What had other feminists had to say on the issue? I wondered.

## Incapable women

If you go back another twenty-odd years from *The Whole Woman* you can find another feminist classic, Adrienne Rich's 1976 seminal text, *Of Woman Born*.[4] Again, the book is not really about birth itself, but addresses the whole package of motherhood. Within it Rich presents childbirth as being entirely taken over by patriarchal forces, and admits that, in spite of her usual propensity to question the status quo, she herself willingly handed over her power and autonomy in birth to the 'experts'. She speculates that this was because she associated passivity with being more womanly, and felt in turn that womanliness was a prerequisite of motherhood. 'I was also, of course, mistrustful of and alienated from my body,' she adds.

Skip forward nearly a quarter of a century to 2011 and you can find Caitlin Moran saying many of the same things. In her feminist bestseller, *How to Be a Woman*,[5] Moran compares her first 'bad birth', with her second 'good birth'. Moran felt she learned to fear birth from her mother, 'returning after delivering every sibling as white as death; hobbling into the house seven times with a bad story'. Like me, she'd planned a home birth with her first; like me, she felt deep down that birth was not physically possible; like me, this doubt was further compounded by going two weeks past her due date. 'I feel like a failed shaman pointing my staff at the sky, shouting, "BEHOLD! THE RAIN!" as the crops continue to wither in the fields,' she writes. Unlike me, her labour did start naturally, but – due to slow progress and a badly positioned baby – she transferred to hospital.

There the midwife who first assessed her told her, 'This is what often happens with the mummies who say they want a home birth . . . they end up having to come in here, and get their tummies cut open.' Like so many women, Moran is not particularly outraged by this attitude, because it rings so deeply true. 'Finally, I have met someone who realizes what I have known all along. This bitch sees me for what I am: incapable.' Her birth was agonising, traumatic, and ended in an emergency caesarean.

I have seen Moran's narrative play out in a thousand birth stories. Women enter into the birth system with a deep lack of confidence in their bodies, and the system then proves to them that they were absolutely right to feel this way. In fact Moran, Rich and

Greer all highlight this same key issue – our tendency to see both women and their bodies as fragile and in need of rescue seems to completely sky-rocket during pregnancy. This, coupled with the disproportionate fear that both women and health care practitioners feel, drives everyone concerned to become complicit in a birth experience in which a woman is most often passive and which is likely to fall somewhere between unpleasant and horrific.

# The set-up

Ever had this conversation?

'How was the birth?'

'Oh, you know, not that great actually. I'd planned for it to be natural, but then my labour went on and on, I was in labour for 38 hours, it was awful, and then, in the end, my plans went out the window, and I had to have forceps/a caesarean.'

It's a familiar tale, and although we may be in the feminist 'fourth wave',* [6] one that nobody seems to question. These are the women who most often feel terrible in the wake of the birth, not just physically, but emotionally. These are the women who so often feel a sense of shame or regret that they 'got their hopes up', that they were foolish enough to have confidence that their bodies would not let them down. And these are the women, as you will discover if you

---

\*      Some see the history of feminism in 'waves'. Put simply: First wave = early twentieth-century suffrage; Second wave = sixties to eighties, equality; Third wave = nineties to noughties, inclusivity; Fourth wave = 2010 to present day, fighting harassment and misogyny, often using technology/social media.

only ask a few more questions, who are victims of a set-up, for in the majority of cases they were not let down by their bodies, but by a system that did not properly support them, and – deeper still – by a culture that accepts and supports that system as something every woman should be grateful for.

You will discover that these women were routinely induced even though they were only a week or so past their due date. You will find that they were turned away from hospital because they 'weren't in labour' and sent home feeling defeated and anxious. You will find that they were left by themselves at times when they needed support. You will hear how they were interrupted, examined, or in some other way made to feel startled, vulnerable, open or exposed, at least once during those hours of 'ineffective' labour. You will find that they remember words that were said to them that might have been meant to reassure, but in fact made them lose confidence in themselves. You will hear how they lay on a bed on their back. You will find that there are a thousand reasons why their bodies did not open as they should and that most of them are due to the environment and circumstances in which they were expected to give birth, the nature of the care and support they received, and that still more of them can even be traced back to the doubt and the negative expectations they already had before they even saw the blue line on the pregnancy test. And you will find, in spite of all this, that they blame themselves.

One solution that's often put forward by midwives and birth experts is for women to reframe the way they think about birth. Learning to believe in yourself and your body's natural abilities, as Caitlin Moran did before her second birth, is a challenge that many women undertake in pregnancy, in Moran's case using the mind-over-matter technique of hypnobirthing. Reframing the pain of birth as positive helped her get through it, 'Unlike all other pain on earth, these don't signal something going wrong but something going right,' she writes of her contractions, adding that the first words she said after her daughter was born were, 'That was easy! Why doesn't anyone tell you it's so easy!'

This, in my experience, is exactly where any feminist dialogue around birth runs into deep and difficult waters. What Moran learned from her 'bad birth' and her 'good birth' – while it may be backed up by the rafts of women whose experiences mirror hers – is highly controversial. The notion that birth can be 'easy', life-enhancing, triumphant, or even pleasurable, and worse still, that the pain of it can be reframed in a positive way, can cause an outcry, one that usually divides women into two entirely fictitious and unhelpful camps, with 'hairy home birthers' on one side and 'too posh to push' on the other. In reality, women are complex and unlikely to be living stereotypes, but the divisive and polarising discussions do serve as a welcome distraction from the real issues, diminishing much hope of our ever collectively improving birth for women of the future.

Changing the way you think is also simply not enough, and can be part of the set-up. Closing your eyes, clicking your heels together three times and saying, 'Pain is power' repeatedly might help, but if you're birthing in a system that doesn't tend to be built with women's physiology in mind, you might be blown off course in spite of your efforts. Added to this, you might actually need medical help – in spite of the many birth affirmations that tell us we need to 'trust birth' because our bodies, 'know what to do', this is not the case for everyone – so feminism also needs to look at how women who can't or don't want to birth naturally or even vaginally, can still be central to decision making and feel like goddesses throughout. Telling women to 'trust birth' without addressing the underlying issues is simply lining them up to fail and, again, has a built-in polarity that helps no one.

## Two doors

Another high-profile feminist, Naomi Wolf, tackles these issues in her 2001 book *Misconceptions*,[7] which, like *The Whole Woman* and *Of Woman Born*, explores birth within the wider context of motherhood and womanhood, rather than as its main focus, as this book aims to do. Wolf writes about 'two doors' – a metaphor that coincidentally echoes my own experience of being referred to the obstetrician who 'believed in vaginal birth', when I could so easily have taken the door into the office of the one who didn't. 'When women start on the journey toward childbirth, most can see only two totally distinct doors available to them: the "conventional" door and the "natural" door,' she writes. Naomi Wolf, who herself had two caesareans, suggests, quite rightly, that bridges need to be built. Each 'door', she argues – the high-tech hospital route and the natural approach – has skills to share with the other: 'Each needs to be talking with the other in a relationship of equality and respect, collaborating with the other, and creating a birth culture and real choices for women out of the best that each has to offer.' But nearly twenty years after Wolf wrote these words, I can vouch for the fact that many of these bridges are yet to be built, with the polarised split in the birth world a long-standing and unresolved problem that works to women's detriment.

In Wolf's native America, this polarisation of birth is extreme, with those who opt for high-tech hospital deliveries likely to be hooked up to a monitor, augmented with a drip, given an epidural and have routine membrane sweeps and their waters broken as standard. As you might expect, a counter-culture of natural birth also exists in the States, with women who want to take the 'alternative' door struggling to find care providers to support them, and even making the choice to birth unassisted rather than enter the highly medicalised system.

Another split ideology is the idea that birthing women are either 'powerful' or 'powerless' and cannot be both. It's true that birth is a huge force that is certainly bigger than us and cannot be fully controlled. It's also true that there is much we can do to maximise our chances of a positive experience. The choices we make in childbirth can and do have an impact on how our birth eventually unfolds, and the idea that we are weak and helpless in the face of the mysterious forces of Mother Nature is yet another myth that discourages women from taking an active role in their birth choices on a daily basis. Neel Shah is an obstetrician and Harvard professor, who is working to change the culture of US labour wards in a bid to reduce their sky-rocketing caesarean rates. 'The biggest factor in whether a woman will have a caesarean delivery,' he writes, 'is the door she walks through to give birth.'[8] Yes, birth can be unpredictable. And, *and*, we have agency.

# ASSERTIVENESS IN MATERNITY CARE

## Know your rights

Be very clear in your own mind that you have the legal and
moral right to be the key decision maker in your maternity care.
You also have the right to be treated with respect and dignity,
and to have full information given to you about any choices
you may need to make. If you feel that your rights are not being
respected, get in touch with one of the support organisations in
the Resources section (see page 311).

## Know what you want

Take time to think about what kind of birth you want and what
elements are important to you. Be flexible in your approach to
planning and think about what you will want in all eventualities,
not just your ideal birth. Once you have made your choices, you
do not need to apologise for them or try to make others feel
better about what you are asking for. Birth is a huge event in your
life and you are entitled to have clear ideas about it. This does
not mean that you are unrealistic, inflexible or demanding. It just
means that you are a strong woman and you believe that you
matter.

## Know why you want it

Look in to the research behind your specific situation – for example, if you are pregnant with twins, or want a VBAC, or are past your due date, or keen on a home birth. Be clear in your own mind what your options are and what you would prefer. Talk to other women (social media is a gold mine for this!) about the choices they made and why they feel these choices were right – or wrong – for them. Being well informed will help you feel more confident in discussions with your care providers.

## Take up space

Have a sense of entitlement – or, if this is something you struggle with, take this opportunity to develop one. Think about your body language in situations in which you need to 'stand up' for yourself. At home by yourself, practise standing tall, feeling grounded and connected to your feet on the floor, drawing back your shoulders and breathing calmly and deeply. Find support if you need to through self-help, therapy, or perhaps yoga and meditation. Developing your confidence and finding your voice will almost certainly help you in your maternity care, and even more so in the next phase of your life – parenthood.

## Build your team

It's much easier to assert yourself when you know you have back-up. If you have a partner or friends who plan to support you in the birth, talk to them about your needs and desires and make sure they are clear about your wishes and totally on side. Find a doula, an independent person who can support you in your birth, and build a relationship with them in which you trust and understand each other. Try to get continuity of care from a midwife if you can, and even if you can't, try to create good, positive connections with your local team of health care providers.

## Vote with your feet

If you feel you are not getting what you want from your care providers, then consider making a move. There may be another hospital or team in your area that you can switch to, and if you are having a planned caesarean, you can travel even further from home to find a care provider who you feel will meet your needs. Your options may differ according to where you are in the world, but there will usually be several to consider. Again, social media is an excellent way to find out what the alternatives are in your local community.

## Use your voice

Say what you want, and don't want, clearly. Practice phrases like, 'I would like more time to consider before I make my decision', 'I don't feel fully informed about that choice, could you say more please', 'I would like you to stop immediately', or 'I do not give my consent to that'. If you feel that your care providers are using unsupportive language or even being disrespectful – tell them. If necessary, make a formal complaint. This will not only help you but also those people who use the maternity service in the future.

## Sorrow and trauma

To say that we are not powerless in birth can be extremely triggering for those women who feel that they absolutely were, and this alone could explain the lack of feminist attention to the birth experience. Such a large percentage of women have had utterly dreadful birth experiences in the past few decades, and they've been given these experiences in a well-rehearsed cultural package bound up neatly with the ribbon of unwavering faith in medical science to rescue them from their inadequate bodies. And the bow on top is the repeated mantra that a healthy baby is all that matters, setting them up for a lifetime of reluctance to question whether their experience could have been less traumatic, could have been different, could even have been glorious.

Anyone who talks about birth in positive terms, therefore, can face a huge backlash, which often seems to me to come from a very hurt place, a wound in women that is often both personal and cultural. I felt the pain of it myself, when, after my first hospital forceps birth, a friend, who had been pregnant at the same time, had the easy home birth that I had been hoping for. I can still remember where I was when I heard the news, and it floored me. I felt gutted – and yes I know that some people will try to tell me that this was simply because I had been set up to view one kind of birth as somehow 'better' than the other, that I felt I had failed the test somehow, and my home birth friend had passed it. But I was not gutted because I had had my silly head filled with unrealistic ideas of the perfect birth – far from it. I was gutted because I was *traumatised*. I hated to think about her birth because it brought up so many 'what if' questions about mine. I was so deeply wounded by my own birth that it was almost unbearable to think that it could have been different for me.

But it could have. It could have been different. I know that now, but it took some painful soul searching, several years, and the birth of another baby to even begin to help me make peace with that fact. I now know that a different 'door', a different midwife, a different cultural backdrop, a different mindset, a different doctor – might have led me to that home birth – or at least to a hospital birth without meeting the obstetrician I affectionately dubbed 'Cutlery Ken'. Humour always helps with trauma, right? It could have been different.

Saying this does not invite yet more polarity. My concluding that some of my own interventions were unnecessary does not mean that *all* interventions are unnecessary. My own desire for home birth does not mean that I desire that choice for every woman. My personal acknowledgement that my birth could have been different, is, for me, about the bigger picture. It's about the future of birth, not the past, although, having said that, in order to move forward, perhaps womankind would benefit from some kind of collective apology? An acknowledgement that it could have been different for all those women who missed their chance for a positive or empowering experience and instead got a birth they would rather forget. And an admission that this was not because their bodies failed them but because they didn't get the empathy-based care they deserved. Who would step up and give this apology? That, I'm less sure about, but women need it, nonetheless. Currently in Western culture there is such a huge lack of acknowledgement for the unnecessary trauma so many women have suffered in birth, and a really strong drive to continue to convince women that it could not have been, and never could be, any other way. This consistently serves to close down dialogue about how to improve birth, and, as feminists, I think it's time to challenge this.

> *The baby is the goal and the how of it is something women are taught belongs to other people to decide. We begin to feel like maybe this is the first real lesson of motherhood – to sacrifice ourselves for the greater good, and express nothing but gratitude for the privilege.*
>
> Clementine Ford[9]

## Lacking attention

When I wrote about the case of Kimberly Turbin's forced episiotomy in a 2014 article for *BestDaily*, I described birth as 'the land that feminism forgot'. I can't help feeling that this was a bit harsh, given the number of writers I've since discovered, particularly in the world of academia, who are taking these topics to beautiful and analytical depths. And, of course, there are leading birth writers and activists – Ina May Gaskin, Sheila Kitzinger, Janet Balaskas and others. But for most people, these voices are off the radar, and the mainstream feminist world is failing to express any particular outrage about what is happening to women in the birth room. In the fourth wave of 'digital feminism', so many vital issues have quite rightly been raised – equal pay, Page 3, FGM, racist and sexist stereotyping, online abuse, everyday sexism – to name just a few. But birth hasn't really made the list.[10] Is this because many of the new generation of activists are yet to become mothers? This may be a factor, but I think the answer goes deeper, to both the collective birth trauma women carry and to the long-standing alignment of feminism with 'equality', and a corresponding reluctance to address issues of feminine biology that set women apart from men, of which birth is of course the prime example. 'One is not born, but rather becomes, a woman,' wrote Simone de Beauvoir in her 1949 classic *The Second Sex*,[11] and this set the tone for much of the feminist discourse ever since, the argument being that patriarchal oppression is built on treating women as the 'other', literally the 'second sex', she-who-is-lacking. Men are the prototype human, and women are this rather odd and dysfunctional afterthought, made from man's spare rib and not very effectively put together at that. 'The female is female by virtue of a certain lack of qualities,' said the charming Aristotle, and de Beauvoir quotes him, quite rightly asserting that this viewpoint has provided the basis for a couple of thousand years of misogyny. However, it's precisely Aristotle's attitude that seems to underpin much of maternity care, and by arguing that birth could be improved, and that the majority of women's bodies work much better than they are currently being given credit for, we are doing something overtly feminist – that is if feminism means celebrating women's bodies as intelligent design, raising women up, and making sure they don't get a raw deal. From

Aristotle to modern maternity care, the idea that women need to be rescued from their lesser, lacking, dysfunctional female forms continues to go unchallenged.

In a world in which feminists have, for a long time, strived for the same privileges that being male affords, the idea that being a woman in itself is something unique and to be celebrated, can also be unfashionable. Within this context, motherhood, breastfeeding, and birth – particularly natural birth – are often devalued and seen as unimportant to the experience of being human. Author Laurie Penny has spoken about her choice not to be a mother at all: 'I can't be bothered,' she writes, and rightly asks why this choice must be questioned, 'Motherhood is a matter of consent,' she says.[12] Another twenty-first-century feminist, Chimamanda Ngozi Adichie, has recently had her first baby, but her concerns – also valid – revolve around the right to maintain a career: 'There are so many women for whom pregnancy is the thing that pushed them down, and we need to account for that. We need to have a clause in every job that a woman who gets pregnant gets her job back in exactly the same way.'[13] Penny and Adichie are concerned with consent and rights, but the birth room itself, where both of these issues are crying out for attention, doesn't get a mention.

Overall, the popular discourse about birth tends to become polarised, with some seeing natural birth, home birth, freebirth (and, often in the same package, breastfeeding and childcare) as the ultimate feminist statement and medicalised birth as oppressive, with others arguing that the complete opposite is the case. Once this argument has gone round the houses a few times, at some point you're bound to hear the refrain, 'Of course, it's all down to personal choice,' and everyone will nod with satisfaction as if the matter is settled. But personal choice is complicated. We all like to think we are making free choices but, of course, we are all a product of our culture, of the stories we have heard, the adverts and TV programmes we have seen, and of the expectations we have therefore built of any given event. If you give birth on a bed on your back, for example, this might feel like a free choice, but there are a myriad of influences – from reality documentaries showing typical hospital birth to the fact that most birth rooms have a fudging great big bed at the centre – that may have influenced you to think that this is 'how birth is done'. Feminism needs to go deeper, and reframe birth choices and experiences within the context of human rights, thereby creating a world in which women's birth choices are much, much broader.

## The cult of natural birth

Some feminist commentators have suggested that women who choose to give birth 'counter-culturally' – for example at home, or using hypnobirthing, water birth, or declining pain relief – are also doing so because of a powerful external influence, this time from 'natural birth advocates,' whom some have gone so far as to describe as an 'industry' or even an 'ideology' or 'cult'. The journalist Hadley Freeman, writing in the *Guardian* in 2015, declared natural birth was 'just another way to judge a woman,' adding that at antenatal classes women were 'berated for opting for a birth plan that involves anything more sophisticated than giving birth in a woodland attended to only by twinkly-eyed foxes'.[14] Eliane Glaser, also writing in the *Guardian* in the same year, described natural birth as a 'cult' that had 'gone too far'. 'Being bullied into natural birth is not what I call feminism,' she stated. The language of her article is pretty extreme: 'Our culture regards natural childbirth as a hazing ritual, a fitting prelude to maternal martyrdom,'[15] she writes. If you don't know what 'hazing' means, as I didn't when I first read her piece, it refers to the often brutal initiation rituals most often favoured by Varsity football players and Ivy League frats, often involving being tied up, beaten, or forced into sex acts.[16] That's quite a comparison.

Hans Peter Dietz, Professor of Obstetrics at the University of Sydney, who is scathing of the current drive to reduce caesarean rates, describes what he calls the 'natural birth ideology' in an interesting way too – he calls it 'paternalism in a skirt'.[17] One implication of Dietz, Glaser, Freeman and all critics of 'physiological' birth is that the women who choose it may have simply replaced their obedience to medical authority in past decades with a new kind of brainwashing; in short, they are under a spell. The clipboard-wielding and patronising doctor may have disappeared, but he has simply been replaced by another leader whom women follow without question – the wholesome antenatal teacher: sandals, chunky jewellery, a waft of neroli oil, perhaps even a floaty dress. However she looks, beware: she is the patriarchy in drag.

Reading these viewpoints is interesting for me, and forces me to revisit my own birth choices. Was I brainwashed in some way, was I under a spell, when I first became interested in the experience of natural birth, and thought, yes, that's what I'd ideally like for myself? I'll admit to reading the birth stories in a book called *Ina May's Guide to Childbirth* and finding them a revelation. Pregnant for the first time, I had only the brutal school video of a woman in a Laura Ashley dress and bug-eyed eighties glasses, lying on her back and having stuff done to her nether regions, as a frame of reference for 'what birth will be like'. The women in Ina May's book gave birth in Gaskin's commune in Tennessee, many of them travelling from all corners of the US to do so, and while they were not all 'hippies,' there's definitely a hippy vibe to Ina May herself who sees labour in psycho-sexual-spiritual terms. In spite of this, the stories in her book were so relatable – these women did not romanticise labour, they still talked about their pain, and their fear, but overwhelmingly to me they came across as women 'just like me,' who felt this pain and fear but who were also tough, in touch with their bodies, sassy, and powerful. I'd never given birth, but I'd pushed through other challenges, and I felt interested in what it might be like to take on the task of labour in a conscious way, with the reward, at least according to the pages of Ina May, being a birth that felt spiritual, ecstatic, empowering, and full of health and strength. At the time of my pregnancy my partner and I used to watch Ray Mears's *Survival* on TV, and whenever I did something particularly resourceful we would joke – with our tongues firmly in our cheeks – that I had 'Rayetta'd it'. And that was my plan for birth. I was going to be one of the tough, capable women I'd read about in Gaskin's book – I was going to Rayetta it. Mears in a skirt, you might even say.

But my birth plans were not entirely built out of the positive and the powerful. My desire to give birth naturally was to some extent about what I wanted, but perhaps even more about what I *didn't* want. I had a deep fear of hospitals, and in particular the scalpels and needles they contained. I hated the idea of a caesarean and was not sure if I could survive being cut open while I was conscious. As someone who fainted when they had a flu jab the idea of an epidural made my blood run cold. So I basically thought, I'm going to do all I can to avoid that. I had no idea what the pain of childbirth was going to be like, but I knew it would have to reach medieval proportions before the idea of a needle in my back seemed like a good plan. I was not fixed in my mindset. I would have been happy to take all the drugs if I'd felt I could no longer Rayetta it. As it turned out, I never got to the point where I felt I couldn't cope, not that it wasn't, at times, unspeakably painful and tough. That birth ended in forceps and this made my physical and emotional recovery difficult, but the next two, both 'hands-off' births, kneeling upright, at home in water, brought home to me one great value of natural birth – that you feel fantastic *afterwards*. I still remember standing on my doorstep in the early September afternoon sunshine after the birth of my third, cradling him in my arms, when a neighbour walked past. She was astounded, literally *flabbergasted*, that I had given birth just a few hours earlier. 'That's impossible!' she cried. 'You look absolutely amazing!' I did, and I felt it too.

Inspiring birth stories, a fear of needles and the desire to impress my neighbours may all have been contributing factors in my choices, but what really influenced me to choose natural birth was evidence. I did my homework. I did what, as a twenty-first-century woman and a graduate, I had done before in many other situations – I read books. I was a birth autodidact – there was no antenatal teacher standing behind me, giving me an Indian head massage and talking about the wonders of my yoni. I went on a solo mission to learn all I could, and I concluded that, while it might not happen for me, a straightforward, physiological, vaginal birth would be my first choice for me and my baby, and that the best way to maximise my chances of getting this was to enter the birth room with a sense of my own rights and power, and to try – if possible – not to step on the 'intervention carousel'.

In my opinion, it's problematic to suggest (perhaps inadvertently) that I, and the hundreds of thousands of women like me who do the same homework and come to the same conclusions are merely cultural sheep, following a trend and wanting to join a special Girls' Club or even a cult, without having given much thought to their motivations. This attitude, that women who want natural birth are brainwashed idiots, can even be dressed up as a feminist viewpoint, with commentators again trotting out the trope that, 'a healthy baby is all that matters'. 'As long as you're both alive and well at the end of childbirth, who cares how you deliver?'[18] wrote Shannon Kyle in a take-down of the NCT in the *Independent* in 2016, while Hadley Freeman concluded her thoughts in the *Guardian* with: 'Childbirth is not a lifestyle statement but a temporary state where the goal is to get out a healthy baby who has a healthy, happy mother to look after it, and whether that's achieved through c-section or by giving birth under a rainbow, then it's all for the good.'

The reason such viewpoints jar with my own feminist principles is not so much because of my own personal experiences or preferences but because of the large numbers of women I speak to every week whose birth trauma is entirely sidelined by such attitudes. These are women who hoped everything would be straightforward, and who indeed ended up alive with a living baby in their arms, but for whom the experience was one in which they felt out of control, disregarded or even violated. How can it be feminist to question their original hopes for a normal birth as 'lifestyle statements,' or dismiss their postnatal anguish because on the surface they seem to be 'healthy'? What we are facing, here in the twenty-first century, is a situation in which grown-up women are being treated with disrespect, coerced into choices, lacking in bodily autonomy, unclear on their rights, receiving shocking postnatal care, not being properly supported or treated during their labours and then getting to carry all of the blame when their bodies 'don't work' properly.

This is an intersectional issue too, for the same is happening to all women, regardless of race, education, or economic background. Indeed, much of the evidence tells us that if you are from a minority group or a poor socio-ecomonic background, you are even *less* likely to have your voice heard in your maternity care. Being a white 'middle-class mummy,' so often used as a derogatory term by health care providers, does at least mean that you have the resources to learn about your options, the confidence to articulate your needs, and no barriers of institutionalised racism to prevent you from being properly listened to. We know from the 2018 MBRRACE-UK[19] report that black women in the UK are five times more likely to die as a result of complications in their pregnancy than their white counterparts. Asian women are nearly twice as likely to die than white women. We know that women in UK prisons are not getting adequate maternity care. We know that women from poorer socio-economic backgrounds have both poorer outcomes and report poorer birth experiences. The picture is the same or worse if we look globally, and the bottom line is always this: women are not being listened to.

To dismiss the voices of women who stand up and say they want and deserve a good birth experience as unimportant or, worse still, whinging, self-centred, and misguidedly obsessed with natural birth to their own detriment, in my opinion completely misses the point. Many women across the board are having birth experiences that damage and distress them. Belittling the ones who dare to raise their voices to complain not only negates their personal value as individuals but also negates the value of *all* women and undermines any attempts to improve birth for the women of the future.

# #metoointhebirthroom

But that was 2015, this is now. Something has happened since, that, although on the surface doesn't seem to relate directly to birth, has still changed everything: #metoo. This huge global conversation about women's bodily autonomy, propelled even further by the behaviour of Weinstein and the subsequent movement of #timesup, is a game changer. This watershed moment in women's feminist history forces us to rethink birth just as it forces us to rethink every other area of our lives. Little ripples of recognition that we might need a #metoointhebirthroom have already begun. In October 2017, as the #metoo movement was just beginning to gather momentum, the UK charity Birthrights stated that, '#metoo shows we need trauma-informed maternity care,' highlighting the need for, 'respectful maternity care that protects human dignity and autonomy' and clarifying that, 'an individual should not need to disclose previous trauma in order to access care that is sensitive to their needs'.[20] They shared two anonymous letters from abuse survivors to birth policy makers, one of whom felt supported in her choice to home birth: 'I never acknowledged at the time that my childhood sexual abuse experiences would have ever had anything to do with how I birthed a baby, but now I can see that they were right at the heart of why I needed to birth how I did. I needed to feel safe to be able to open, both physically and emotionally, and I needed people around me who trusted in the birth process, and in me . . . No one had put anything inside me, none of my negative memories had been triggered and I had a wholly positive birth experience leaving me feeling like I could do anything.' The other letter was from a woman who had also planned a home birth but had what she describes as a 'very typical NHS birth': 'For the whole pregnancy and during birth,' she wrote, 'a woman is expected to open her legs, over and over again, and have many people touching her genitals, and she is expected to just get on with it all like a good girl and do it with a smile, while those people insert their hands and/or instruments inside her, sometimes roughly, or stand around talking between themselves while she lies down with her legs wide open . . . Looking back honestly and without trying to sweeten it for myself, it was one of the most impersonal and humiliating experiences I have endured as an adult . . . I'm tired of saying it was OK just because me and my baby survived and that we should be grateful it wasn't worse.'

Given how widespread we know that sexual abuse, rape, and violations of women's body boundaries are – and arguably we are still only just beginning to get a sense of this – many more conversations about autonomy and agency in the birth room are urgently needed. But not only, as Birthrights point out, should we not expect women to disclose abuse to professionals in their maternity care, we should also be treating *all* women with kindness, dignity, respect and empathy *as standard*. 'Special treatment' should be for everyone. There's a wider connection between #metoo and consent in the birth room that applies to every interaction between birthing woman and care provider, not just those that may seem openly disrespectful. As #metoo is only just beginning to fully highlight, one person may be happy in an interaction and consider it normal or even fun, while the other may be silently suffering. More empathy for women's experiences, in birth and every other situation, is needed right now in our culture.

> *Wherever in society there is a power imbalance, there is a lack of empathy. Somebody powerful has forgotten to ask, 'What is this like for you?' We need to start building empathy, and we need to start building it everywhere.*
>
> Deborah Frances-White (commenting on #metoo)[21]

If women begin truly to voice their discontent, and say 'this is what it was like for me,' then this will surely help in the construction of empathy; there is huge power in storytelling. But, for a long time, women have tended to be discouraged from talking about their birth experiences, as Eva Wiseman pointed out in the *Guardian* in April 2018: 'Many of us approach it with a certain horror, having never seen or heard the many truths of what we're heading for, and one grim effect of that is that we have no idea of our place in the room, other than birthing object that something happens to. Surely there are a thousand #metoo moments happening in delivery rooms across the country, in part due to pregnant women's ignorance and fear. We don't know what's right, which means that, also, we don't know what's wrong.'[22] Wiseman is correct that women often don't know what's right, but they certainly *do* know what's wrong, because, like all violations, it *feels* wrong, and it's always felt wrong. The current wave of feminism, epitomised by #metoo, is suddenly emboldening women to speak out about experiences that have felt wrong to them for decades, and this collective shift in consciousness is beginning to reach pregnant and birthing women, too. Writing about her birth experiences in March 2018, New York-based journalist Justine van der Leun describes how, when she pressed her obstetrician for answers about how her high-risk pregnancy might impact on her professional life, he became irritable, accusing her of 'only caring about her work'. At this moment, she suddenly felt the power imbalance of their interaction in a new way: 'I am not a woman who shies away from conflict and have never once been mistaken for a people-pleaser,' she writes. 'But had this interaction occurred two years earlier, I would have experienced a furtive rush of fear, convinced that I was at the man's mercy. For the sake of my baby, I would have told myself, I would do well to yield, to calm him, to agree, to defuse – and then to go home and privately rage, feeling young and dumb and female. But now I saw the situation from the outside, through the lens of the feminist uprising that saturated the news. From this view, a woman was sitting on the examination table, the specialist standing before her. He was up, she was down. He was the expert, she the civilian. He had recently been elbow-deep inside her. Each time they met, only one of them was carrying a baby they could lose. And only one of them was wearing pants.'[23] Each and every woman experiencing maternity care right now needs to allow #metoo to reach into her birth room experience in this way.

It is a powerful revelation to realise that – in spite of your pregnancy – you still matter, just as you did before you conceived, and just as you will after your baby is born. This may seem like it should go without saying, but we need to bear in mind a long history of seeing pregnant women as 'vessels,'[24] mere containers for the baby and by this implication as disposable as any other form of packaging. Enforced caesareans have happened on UK soil[25] and globally, and in a world that is usually very careful to gain consent for organ donation, we might argue that this renders pregnant women with less bodily autonomy than a corpse. In Ireland, the recently repealed Eighth Amendment, a piece of legislation that gives equal right to life to the unborn as it does to the mother, has had disastrous effect in the cases of women like Savita Halappanavar,[26] who lost her life when she was denied life-saving treatment during a miscarriage, but also continues to creep into the Irish delivery room. One woman who gave birth there in 2015 said to me, 'They told me, "You will give birth when, how and where we decide." When I questioned their decisions they said, "Clearly someone has to be the voice for your baby since you are not being very rational."' And in a myriad of small ways, from being made to birth in positions that don't feel comfortable, to being mocked for attempts to take control of their birth, to being talked into choices they don't feel happy with, pregnant women's autonomy and freedom is infringed constantly, all around the world.

We need to open our eyes and challenge this cultural backdrop, which subtly but surely impacts on an individual pregnant woman's sense of entitlement, or lack of it – just as having a man in the White House who talks about 'grabbing women by the pussy,'[27] and concludes after the sexual assault testimony of Christine Blasey Ford that it's a 'very scary time for young men in America,'[28] has an impact on every woman's personal sense of autonomy and worth. 'I did try to complain at the time about what happened to me,' a pregnant woman told me as I wrote this chapter, 'but all that happened was they gave me a basic explanation of the rationale behind the procedures I had, and nobody seemed to want to actually listen to my personal experience and why I found it so damaging. Now, a couple of years later, I feel it's probably too late to complain.' Her words echo the story of Blasey Ford and of so many stories from the #metoo movement, too: 'At the time, I tried to report it but nobody listened and my experience was belittled. Now, it's happened too long ago and nobody will believe me.'

So much has changed since I lay on that beach in my twenties, a beer in one hand and Greer in the other. For me personally, I've thought, written, read, loved, lost and wondered for nearly two decades. I've become a mother three times over. Now I'm raising two girls and a boy in a world that keeps rapidly changing, so fast that in the space of just a few months we can suddenly see everything that's wrong with the whole of our living memory and totally rethink it. It's both a thrill to be a part of this world and a sorrow too, as I start to wonder, what did I miss, what did these shackles – that I only just became aware of – prevent me from doing, feeling, knowing and experiencing? It's time to turn this bright, harsh, revealing spotlight on birth, and see it for what it is; an issue not just of women's freedom, autonomy, and agency, but of unnecessarily imposed limits on their power and joy. The feminist conversation has, to date, only fleetingly dipped into a woman's experience of birth, and those feminists who have given birth a mention have had their words quickly forgotten. I've been told before that birth is considered a 'niche issue' by the media, even though every single human is born, and at least 80 per cent of women will directly experience it. 'It is only one day,' we are urged, even though most of us will remember every detail of that day for the rest of our lives. It's time we refused to have the importance of birth diminished – birth matters, and it's in urgent and overdue need of feminist attention.

# Chapter 3

# When Women's Bodies Became Men's Business: A History of Birth

*There is no doubt that the history of childbirth can be viewed as a gradual attempt by man to extricate the process of birth from woman and call it his own.*

Suzanne Arms, *Immaculate Deception*[1]

Looking back over the history of birth, it's hard to see it, at least in places, in any terms other than a takeover, and a pretty hostile one at that. The birth room itself seems to be a crucible for a centuries-old power struggle, in which a tug-of-war over who gets the ultimate credit for bringing life into the world is still being played out today. Women who have a positive experience of birth will almost always talk about it in terms of 'power' or 'empowerment' – 'I felt so strong, like I could do anything', is the phrase I hear most often. When women's faces glow as they tell you what a powerful and transformative life experience they have had, you do start to wonder if there is some kind of widespread ongoing patriarchal attempt to tame, diminish, reduce or take ownership of this power. Maybe there's even an envy of it – in a world in which men get the biggest and best slice of the pie in almost every area, birth is, after all, one of the few things they will never be able to experience or possess for themselves. The next best option is to control it, and bask in as much of the reflected glory as they can.

Let's explore the history of this takeover, but before we do, two things need to be said. The first is that some of mankind's attempts to control birth have brought advantage; life-saving developments that benefit women and their babies globally. The second is that, while research tells us that most women prefer physiological birth, it also tells us that those who cannot, or who simply don't wish to give birth naturally, also feel that being in control and central to decisionmaking is key to their having a positive experience.[2] Nevertheless, as we look at the history, much of which concerns the advent of different interventions, we need to be brave enough to question how much our modern levels of interference in birth are helpful to women, and look for balance between the safety they can bring and the detrimental effects they may have on women's experience. Because if you talk to women who felt ecstatic, empowered, and truly triumphant in the aftermath of childbirth, those women have almost always given birth naturally, and on their own terms. We may associate power with money, status or authority – 'We have no template for what a powerful woman looks like, except that she looks rather like a man,' writes Mary Beard in *Women and Power*[3] – but if you have been a woman or been present for a woman who is birthing her baby with little or no interference, you might beg to differ.

I asked a group of women on social media to describe their feelings about their natural births. 'Nobody coached me or touched me or my baby as she emerged – we did it all ourselves, and it felt so wonderful, like I could climb ten mountains and wrestle grizzly bears. I've never felt so fierce and strong and shining in love,' Samantha Norman told me. 'I surrendered into the most powerful thing my body has ever done,' said Katy Beale from London. 'I roared like a lioness and felt like a queen,' added Millie Davis. 'I felt immensely powerful and like I could achieve anything because I had done what everybody told me I could not,' said Jen Higgins from Lancashire. I don't think it's a coincidence that many of these women birthed their babies at home, and in water. Being 'on your own turf' helps hugely to right the currently skewed power dynamic, for in our own homes we are more naturally in the role of 'permission giver,' and any visiting health professional must play the part of 'permission seeker,' whereas this is most often vice versa in hospital: to use a basic example, think, 'Can I use the toilet?' At a hospital birth, it is the woman who must ask this question; at home, it is the midwife or anyone else who steps into the woman's space. Likewise, the birth pool, which as a 'circle full of water' always seems to me to be hugely symbolic of the feminine: the woman is quite literally 'in her element'. The water of the pool, which has also been described as 'the big dark skirts,' automatically gives a woman privacy, freedom of movement and control. And put simply, if you want to touch or see her vagina, you will definitely have to ask first, and you may have to get wet!

We then have to ask ourselves why these immensely powerful experiences of home birth, water birth, and 'hands-off' birth, where a woman is left undisturbed and even 'catches her own baby,' are the hardest types of birth to experience in our culture. If there is a 'cult of natural birth,' it doesn't appear to be very effective: the number of women who actually have a birth that is truly free of any intervention is minuscule. In a game of Birth Intervention Bingo, many readers of this book would get a line, if not a full house. Have a go!

| Induction | Membrane Sweep | Waters Broken Artificially | Syntocinon Drip |
|---|---|---|---|
| Electronic Monitoring | Told When to Push | Epidural | Instrumental Delivery |
| Feet in Stirrups | Injection for Placenta | Caesarean | Opioids |
| Episiotomy | Gas and Air | Routine Vaginal Exams | Antibiotics |

Birth interventions are 'marketed' as being in the name of safety, and we know that in many cases, they are necessary and life-saving. However, the world's most prestigious health journal, *The Lancet*, has highlighted that women in high-income countries are likely to experience a 'too much too soon' approach to their care, with the detrimental over-application of routine interventions.[4] We also know that interventions such as caesarean[5] and induction[6] continue to rise rapidly and in disproportion to improvements in birth outcomes, and that they vary greatly according to geography,[7] both of which suggest that many women are having high-intervention births when they don't actually need them. Even births that are currently considered 'normal,' 'straightforward' or even 'natural' tend to contain some interventions; a woman or midwife may describe a birth in this way if there has been an artificial induction, continuous monitoring, or even forceps. A report from the Royal College of Midwives in 2016 found that, while the rate of 'normal births' is recorded at around 65 per cent, further analysis which asked more questions about the exact interventions each birth involved reduced that figure to around 20 per cent.[8]

One in five? How have we ended up here? It seems like we have completely lost sight of what birth 'is' or what it 'could be' – and we are now in a place where the type of birth that would have once seemed alarmingly medicalised is now our only frame of reference for 'normality'. Normal birth has somehow become 'abnormal,' a strange and risky choice that only a minority can or do make, with a well-known adage of obstetricians being that 'birth is only normal in retrospect'. In other words, all birth must be assumed *abnormal* until it is over. In this framework, the term 'normal birth' has itself become problematic, mostly because nobody really can agree on what it means any more, and because so few women are getting it that it has been deemed exclusive or even shaming terminology. To say some births are 'normal' implies that others must be 'abnormal' and is hurtful to anyone whose birth did not meet the criteria for 'normal' – which is currently the vast majority of women.

Terminology like 'positive birth' or 'enjoyable birth' is perhaps more helpful, as it cuts through the polarities. Positive birth experiences can encompass births with all available medical interventions or none, and everything in between. However, many women are not having a positive or enjoyable birth either and are instead left with a range of feelings from disappointed to traumatised but unable to challenge what happened to them. They feel disempowered, but it can be socially unacceptable to complain about your birth – in fact when I spoke to another group of women on social media about their traumatic births, most of them wished to be anonymous, perhaps a sign of this taboo. Often, these vitally important voices, that teach us so much about what matters, are left unheard. 'I felt disempowered, like a child, humiliated as people barked and laughed at me, all my requests ignored and unanswered. Like I wasn't there any more, wasn't a person. Then I was handed a baby, like someone had just popped to the shops for one. I felt no connection between this baby and the bump I'd been growing,' said one. 'I remember feeling like I didn't matter at all, only the baby mattered,' said another. Several women described feeling dehumanised: 'After my daughter's birth I felt violated. Empty. Shell-shocked. Like I hadn't really been in the room as a person, but as some kind of dummy,' said one, while another commented, 'I feel it was done *to* me, all control was taken away from me. I was a piece of meat on a conveyor belt.' One described how she felt as if she had been raped, and that she then wrote thank you letters to her care providers in a way that she compares to 'Stockholm syndrome' – the psychological condition in which hostages develop positive feelings towards their captors as a survival strategy.

# The hammer of witches

The idea that birth can be empowering rather than traumatic has in recent times been called a 'Goddess myth,'[9] but to understand how we have arrived in this place, we have to go back, right back, to the Goddess culture, a time, thousands of years ago, when some believe that the 'divine feminine' was given much more spiritual and cultural importance. Then came Christianity, with no female deities and worship of the 'Father and Son' at the centre, and although Mary and the many female saints remained as a nod in the divine feminine's direction, they were never allowed to be worshipped. It was this patriarchal religion that sought to stamp out what it referred to as 'witches' between the fourteenth and sixteenth centuries. In well-organised and funded campaigns, reaching their height in the mid-sixteenth century, Church and State came together to torture and burn what historians have estimated to be millions of people – of which around 85 per cent are believed to have been women and children.

A book called the Malleus Maleficarum – the 'Hammer of Witches' – was published in 1487 by Heinrich Kramer and Jacob Sprenger, and this book became an authoritative and bestselling volume on witchcraft, with detailed information on how to identify, torture and exterminate witches. Those who were accused were most commonly stripped naked, shaved of their body hair, tortured, starved and beaten, and encouraged to name their accomplices before being put to death. And who were these women? Most commonly they would be the local 'wise woman,' older, single or widowed, skilled in healing herbs and remedies, and called upon to help at times of illness, birth and death. In other words, many of those burned were midwives.[10]

Against a church doctrine of 'God in charge,' anyone who took an active role in healing, birth or death was seen as in some way trying to interfere with God's plan and usurp His divine power. 'No one does more harm to the Catholic faith than midwives,' said the authors of the Malleus Maleficarum, who also stated, 'When a woman thinks alone, she is evil.' Our modern misogynistic sense of woman as 'vessel' or 'host' for the fetus may have its roots in the religious belief at this time that, during sex, a fully formed little person or 'homunculus' is deposited in the mother, who simply houses it for the pregnancy until it is born. This idea of a teeny weeny person shooting into our uterus would be pretty funny if it didn't contain within it a real diminishment of women's humanity and personhood. This reduction of women to walking incubators, along with suspicion and discomfort around pregnancy and those who serve pregnant women that often accompanies it, can be a blank slate for persecution, both ancient and modern. Just look at the echoes of this attitude in the words of two different twenty-first-century US representatives as they make their case against the right to termination of pregnancy:

*I understand that they feel like that is their body. I feel*
*like it is a separate – what I call them is, is you're a*
*'host.' And you know when you enter into a relationship*
*you're going to be that host and so, you know, if you*
*pre-know that then take all precautions and don't get*
*pregnant. So that's where I'm at. I'm like, 'hey, your*
*body is your body and be responsible with it. But after*
*you're irresponsible then don't claim, well, I can just go*
*and do this with another body, when you're the host and*
*you invited that in.'*

Oklahoma State Representative
Justin Humphrey, 2017[11]

*It's a complex issue because one has to think, well*
*there's a host body and that host body has to have a*
*certain amount of rights because at the end of the day*
*it is that body that carries this entire other body to*
*term. But there is an additional life there.*

Florida State Representative Jose Oliva, 2019[12]

Prior to and during the witch hunts of the medieval period, another profession arose and took hold: that of the physician. Medical schools sprang up across Europe, and this predominantly male role largely disassociated itself from birth initially, as well as from surgery or any form of dissection that might have led to a better understanding of the workings of the body. Male doctors, who practised medicine largely in the upper classes, used methods such as leeches and bloodletting, and based their approach on the concept of the 'four humours,' in contrast to the understanding of herbalism developed by 'witches'. Yet it was the doctors whose methods gained credibility, largely thanks to the backing of Church and State. Women healers, on the other hand, were widely discredited. 'If a woman dare to cure without having studied she is a witch and must die,' says the Malleus Maleficarum, neglecting to mention that women were barred from such studies.

All of this persecution was not the end of the midwife, but it was certainly an early example of the ongoing wrestle for power in the birth arena, and reflected wider attempts to establish the patriarchal upper hand in every area of life. Essentially, an extensive PR campaign had been successful: the men were established as the scientific experts, and the women were relegated to 'old wives'. This polarised split – the legacy of which we still have today – did nobody any favours; as Adrienne Rich points out, 'The waste of female lives through these centuries was partly avoidable; mortality of both sexes, and from all causes, was high before the discovery of asepsis and the refinement of anatomical knowledge with dissection. But much of it was avoidable, if we remember that a pregnant woman, a woman in labour, is not usually suffering from disease. The midwives' ignorance of progress in medicine and surgery, on the one hand, and the physicians' ignorance of female anatomy and techniques relating to childbirth, on the other, were not inevitable, they were the consequences of internalised misogyny.'[13] If both 'sides' had listened to and learned from each other, history may have been very different.

## Tools of the trade

While birth continued to be a largely all-female event, midwives around the sixteenth and seventeenth centuries began to occasionally call for help from the 'barber surgeons' – men who were, to put it bluntly, tooled up and ready to either deliver your baby or give you a short back and sides. From the barber surgeons came a selection of instruments, helpful and destructive in equal measure, either accidentally causing damage or in many cases saving the life of the mother by dismembering an obstructed baby. The most notable of these, the forceps, has an interesting history indeed.

Invented by barber surgeon Peter Chamberlen in the early seventeenth century, the forceps bring us yet another tale of power and control in the birth room. Kept hidden in a huge and ornately gilded wooden box, so heavy that two men would be needed to carry it to a birth room, the tools were both a money-maker and a closely guarded secret. Used behind locked and guarded doors to deliver obstructed babies at the high price of around £5,000 in today's money, their design – which presumably could have saved many lives of women and babies – was kept totally secret for several generations of Chamberlen men in the sole name of financial profit. Eventually, in 1693, a Chamberlen descendant sold the concept to a surgeon in Holland, but once the cash had been handed over it emerged this was a swindle and only one blade of the forceps was in the box. In a final twist to the tale, the original Chamberlen forceps – long thought to be lost – turned up in the nineteenth century in a box under the floorboards of a house, where, hidden away by Chamberlen's wife, they had remained for a hundred and thirty years.

Once the Chamberlen forceps single blade was out in the public domain, however, other barber surgeons guessed at the full design, and this changed the course of birth forever. Banned from use by women, forceps were used more and more to expediate birth, with one surgeon in the 1880s boasting that he never let women suffer labour until fully dilated before using them, a technique which could cause fatal haemorrhage. This trigger-happy approach was not uncommon – even as late as 1920 a surgeon in America, Joseph DeLee, introduced what he called the 'prophylactic forceps operation' as standard in all births. The result? DeLee made a fortune and every woman in receipt of his method got a large episiotomy and their baby pulled out ASAP, whether they needed it or not.

Chamberlen and DeLee were some of the first to see that where there was a labouring woman, there was money to be made. This was the beginnings of the obstetrics industry we know today, best high-lighted by Ricki Lake and Abby Epstein in their 2008 documentary 'The Business of Being Born,'[14] which pointed out the huge influence of drug companies on the individual experiences of birthing women in the USA. The billion-dollar industry of drugs like the labour augmenting 'pitocin,' they argued, was robbing women of their power and turning them into medical patients at a moment where they ought to be upright, empowered , and experiencing their female strength. I asked Ricki and Abby what they thought had changed for birth in the USA in the decade or so since the film's release: 'Though the film has helped bring about a major consciousness shift and launched a movement that expanded options for women in specific areas, it continues to be a struggle to access midwifery care for many women,' they told me. 'It's very discouraging to see the maternal mortality rate rising, especially among women of colour. In Manhattan, where much of 'The Business of Being Born' was filmed, the last in-hospital birth centre recently closed to accommodate more private rooms. So you still see business as a driving force behind the lack of childbirth options.'

This prioritising of profit in the birth room really began with forceps. Where doctors would normally have only got involved in births that were 'going wrong,' most often to use tools to dismember the baby as this was the only hope of survival for the mother, forceps gave them something seemingly useful to do – and get paid for – in every birth they attended. This single invention brought doctors firmly into the obstetric arena, and these 'men-midwives' lost no time in pushing their female counterparts to the side. Forceps use was also a key prompt in the introduction of the 'lithotomy' position for birth – on your back with your feet held up high or supported. Rendering the birthing woman entirely passive, with the attendents view of her reducing down to a birthing vagina rather than a whole person, nevertheless it makes it much easier for the instruments to be used.

Midwives protested against these changes, most notably Elizabeth Nihell in 1760, who can only be described as a feminist and possibly the very first birth activist. In her *Treatise on the Art of Midwifery*,[15] she labelled the male midwives, 'broken barbers, tailors or pork butchers,' and spoke powerfully against those she felt were profiteering at the expense of the safety of women and babies. Men, with their lesser knowledge and experience, were taking over in the birth room, she protested, and, 'Those poor instruments of God's making, the women's fingers, would not much better and much safer, do everything that is pretended to be done by that same boasted instrument' – the forceps. She also suggested that birth should not be rushed, and that if Nature takes a longer time, she has, 'no doubt a very good reason'. 'Art should aim at imitating Nature; now Nature proceeds leisurely, instead of which the forceps goes too quick to work,' she wrote. On top of all this, she urged readers to listen to the voice of the birthing woman, and, perhaps most remarkably, described a scenario familiar in birth rooms to this day, in which patience is lost with Mother Nature by the woman and those who attend her, the woman is in pain and just wants it over with, the man-midwife applies his instruments, and,

> *Then it is, that in full chorus the deluded parties, in the innocence of their heads and hearts, hold up their hands to heaven, and piously exclaim, 'What a narrow escape the patient had, thanks to the learned Doctor, and what a mercy it was she had not been trusted to such an ignorant creature as a midwife must be.'*
>
> Elizabeth Nihell[16]

The birth wars do indeed have deep roots. Deep, too, are the roots of our feelings about birth interventions, apparently leaving women both ancient and modern with nagging questions: Could we have waited longer? Did that need to happen? Were lives just saved? Should I be grateful to this doctor? Or should I resent him?

*At the time I felt included in decision making. It wasn't until afterwards I realised I was part of the conveyor belt process and the only options provided were those that fitted their timescales without any suggestion of alternatives. My memories are of the midwife filling in paperwork rather than emotional and physical support.*

Gem, Somerset, twenty-first-century birth

*I felt controlled and bullied into having things done that I didn't want to happen. I knew they didn't need to happen but when I had a midwife and a doctor insisting 'it's hospital policy,' I felt powerless, like I had no choice, that my voice didn't matter, that my choices and wishes for my baby's birth were worthless.*

Charlotte Keyworth, West Yorkshire,
twenty-first-century birth

Elizabeth Nihell died in a workhouse and was buried in a pauper's grave, while William Smellie, the obstetrician she was mainly criticising in her treatise, lived a rich and successful life and has come to be considered the 'father of British midwifery,' so it's not difficult to see who won that particular battle. Eighteenth-century birth rooms were more and more often attended by both doctor and midwife, and the entourage of women attendants known as the 'godsibs' or 'gossips,' who had traditionally supported, nurtured, fed and massaged the labouring woman, were banished. While birth, for now, remained at home, it was nevertheless transformed by these steps into a dynamic we would be more familiar with in the present day. An all-female, social and even celebratory event became instead a woman attended by medical experts with whom she had little or no relationship. And as part of this new and more medicalised way of birthing, another divisive and thoroughly modern issue came to the fore: pain.

## Eve's curse

*Unto the woman He said, 'I will greatly multiply thy sorrow and thy conception. In sorrow thou shalt bring forth children; and thy desire shall be to thy husband, and he shall rule over thee.'*

Genesis 3:16

The idea that birth pain or 'Eve's Curse' is God's punishment for women is just one element of this neat little Bible verse, which has also been used as the justification for marital rape. Just as medieval women were persecuted for their attempts at healing which were seen as interference in God's plan, so were they also brought to book for any form of pain-relieving herbs for labour which would likewise represent a challenge to the punishment the Almighty was so keen to bestow on womankind. In contrast, nineteenth-century doctors began to explore the use of both ether and chloroform on labouring women, whose pain was presumably considerably increased by labouring in the lithotomy position and the widespread use of forceps: creating a product to fix the problem you caused yourself is an ingenious piece of marketing if ever there was one. Once again, the Bible was used to justify this move: had not God put Adam into a 'deep sleep' when He removed his rib? they argued. And wasn't man's intelligence in discovering the effectiveness of drugs, in itself, a God-given power? The world seemed ready to accept this new way of thinking, but it was Queen Victoria's use of chloroform in her own labours that really sealed the deal. Just as now we look to Kate Middleton and Meghan Markle for both fashion and birth inspiration, upper-class women in both the UK and the USA were keen to have the same royal experience, which became known as chloroform 'a la reine'.

It's worth talking a little bit about labour pain itself at this point. What is the point of it? Why do we have it? And should we seek to eliminate it? Some argue, 'You wouldn't have a tooth out without pain relief, would you?' and if you think about birth as a 'medical extraction' then this argument stands up pretty well. However, labour pain is different. Birth is not something 'going wrong' with the body, which needs to be numbed, nor is it something horrible being done to you, like the removal of a tooth. Birth is something right, healthy and powerful, the perfect expression of a body at the peak of its powers, and something that is not 'done to' women, but that they do themselves. The argument against being anaesthetised for it is that, not only will you miss out on the human experience itself, but that the drugs themselves may bring other problems, such as side-effects for you[17] and the baby,[18] interference with the production of your own labour hormones,[19] a higher chance of intervention,[20] difficulties with bonding or breastfeeding,[21] and negative long-term effects either from the interventions themselves, for example pelvic floor issues,[22] or from the drug, for example nerve damage caused by epidural.[23] Ina May Gaskin writes that labour pain is 'clean' – when it's over, it's over. 'When avoidance of pain becomes the major emphasis of childbirth care, the paradoxical effect is that more women have to deal with pain *after* their babies are born,'[24] she points out. Most women who choose to attempt labour without pain relief do so with this in mind; they want to stay active and mobile, work with their own body's needs, allow the natural production of hormones to help labour progress well, reduce their chance of interventions, and protect their baby from any possible ill effects. After all, they have spent an entire pregnancy avoiding alcohol, medication and even blue cheese in the name of their baby's healthy development!

And could this pain have a purpose? If you've ever felt the white heat of a contraction, you might already be clenching your fists right now and fantasising about pummelling me in the ovaries for even suggesting such a thing. Giving birth really *really* hurts, for most women, myself included. Some, usually through some kind of powerful mental reframing, experience the sensations as powerful or even erotic – but they're in the minority. From an evolutionary point of view, the sharpness of contractions may have been a signal to women to 'get somewhere safe'. But there's more to it – pain in labour also plays a role in the cocktail of hormones produced. Just as you might find your Saturday 5k run fairly agonising, but feel brilliant afterwards thanks to the endorphins produced from this painful exertion, so too with childbirth. Some studies have found that women report either high[25] or lowered[26] feelings of 'satisfaction' after birth under epidural – although there appear to be no studies on feelings of triumph, achievement, elation and pride after birth – either with or without pain relief. Many women do report feeling it's important to them to be central to the experience of birth, however, and some of the 'dissatisfaction' with epidural birth does come from this need – one study found that around a third of women reported disliking the loss of sensation, and feeling 'robbed' and 'cheated' and that they had not 'participated' or 'contributed' to the labour.[27] Childbirth educator Penny Simkin makes the distinction between 'pain' and 'suffering' in birth, with pain being an unpleasant physical sensation that can be associated with damage, but also with physical exertion, while suffering is a sense of being overwhelmed and help-less. 'Many women suffer in childbirth because they are not kindly treated, they are not respected, they feel unloved, they feel alone,' she says. 'That can turn the pain into suffering. No woman should suffer in childbirth – if she crosses the line to suffering then – we've failed her.'[28] When you put this comment alongside the history of birth we've been exploring in this chapter, it rings especially true, given that what we've essentially seen is labouring women being slowly alienated from their support, their birth room emptying of sisters, mothers and wise women, skilled from experience of many other births and knowledgeable in the many ways of helping and bringing comfort. Such support, we know from several high-quality modern studies,[29] makes the need for birth interventions much less likely, and reduces the need for pain relief.[30] Instead, women have been laid on their back and attended by doctors with tools – men who initially knew very little about the female body and who were for a large part of the eighteenth and nineteenth centuries discouraged from even looking at a woman's genitals. Even in modern times, the expectation to give birth 'naturally' without any drugs may indeed be unrealistic, if everything else about birth stays the same in terms of lack of continuous support, limited mobility, not much knowledge of alternative comfort measures and an environment that feels alien or fearful. There is more to 'natural birth' than simply declining the drugs – we need to start thinking about 'natural' in terms of what a woman truly needs, rather than just being about what she abstains from.

# All or nothing: the angel in the birth room

Some modern feminist commentators have condemned what they see as a current 'trend' for 'natural birth' – which in this context usually translates as 'without pain relief' – arguing that 'nature' is not the kindly mother figure some may cast her as, but rather a cruel and indiscriminate force. Alison Phipps in *The Politics of the Body*[31] argues that 'normal birth' is just part of a modern-day 'middle-class' package of competitive and '*intensive motherhood*,' 'an experience which allows women to find and fulfil themselves through self-sacrifice'. In this narrative, she writes, 'withstanding the ordeal of childbirth is the route to authentic motherhood'. In October 2017 the cover story of *Time*, by Claire Howorth, called this the 'Goddess myth,'[32] essentially, 'that she is built to build a human, that she will feel all the more empowered for doing so as nature supposedly intended and that the baby's future depends on it'. This 'myth,' argues Howorth, has become a vision of perfect motherhood that is unobtainable, and a stick to beat us with. Similarly Elizabeth Badinter, author of *The Conflict*, sees an obsession with 'nature' as a modern phenomenon: 'For me, the epidural was a victory over pain. But they say no, they want to *feel* what it is to be a woman. Their idea is that if you're not suffering you have failed the experience of maternity. You are a "denatured woman".'

In my opinion the naturally birthing woman has become almost a caricature, conceived always as white, middle-class, floaty-dressed, clutching a birth plan and serenely hypnobirthing her way through contractions she will only refer to as 'surges'. Underneath the calm exterior lies a control freak, whose only motivation for enduring this extreme trial is to affirm herself as the ultimate mother, which has become equated with martyrdom. She is reminiscent of the heroine of the Victorian narrative poem, 'The Angel in the House,'[33] a paragon of sweet and submissive womanhood, torn apart by Virginia Woolf in a feminist essay in 1931.[34] 'She was utterly unselfish . . . She sacrificed herself daily. If there was chicken, she took the leg; if there was a draught she sat in it.' This unobtainable image of perfection, that hovers behind us, whispering in our ears of our inadequacy and failure, must, according to Woolf, be 'killed' if we ever want to be creative, authentic beings, although, she adds, 'It is far harder to kill a phantom than a reality.' As women, I think we all need to work together to destroy this idealistic fantasy, this 'Angel in the Birth Room'. One of the best ways of doing this is by telling each other our own authentic stories, because their complexity in itself will destroy this polarised 'shadow,' which is merely a projection on a wall and does not do justice to birthing women's many and various choices, motivations and desires.

Nor must we continue to mock women by referring to their attempts to birth and parent in the best way they can with terms that imply they are trying too hard. 'Intensive motherhood'? As a parent of three young children, I do wish someone would enlighten me about how it could ever *not* be 'intense' – the love, the endless menial tasks, the emotional dynamics, the spilt drinks, the havoc wreaked on my body, my sleep, my bank balance, my Saturday night plans: it seems pretty intense to me. Did I birth without drugs and breastfeed simply because I saw motherhood as a contest that I wanted to win? I wonder why our female motivations must be framed in these terms? My dad, no longer with us, worked seventy-seven hours a week in an off-licence, and even night shifts in a petrol station, to put me through the private school he – rightly or wrongly – felt would give me the best advantage. Did anyone accuse him of martyrdom? I don't recall his choices ever being scrutinised – he was just seen as a 'good man,' 'hard-working,' 'doing the best for his child'. Natural birth or elective caesarean; epidural or hypnosis, bottle or breast – it really is time to stop giving every choice a woman makes a negative spin.

Of course, my dad's herculean efforts did at least buy me a place in the 'middle class' – a term which in recent times seems to have become something of a slur. To me, it means I have privilege and opportunities denied to many, including all previous generations of my family. And it means that when I came to give birth, as with so many other situations in my life, I was lucky to have the educational level that enabled me to research, read, question and understand my options. Shouldn't this opportunity be something that feminists are fighting for all women to have, rather than mocking those that do, as 'middle-class birthzillas'. Such women are so well-informed that they even have the audacity to suggest their care-givers refrain from giving them unnecessary interventions, apparently. Well, I was one such woman. My expectations were well and truly high, my sense of entitlement and worth was positively disruptive. Thanks, Dad.

# 'A night dropped out of my life'

Nobody makes choices in a vacuum, and birth choices, such as the decision to decline or accept pharmacological pain relief, is a response to the kind of birth that is considered normal at any given time in our history, rather than a necessary or unnecessary part of birth itself. In other words, birth pain may be more manageable for some women in some situations than it is in others, and we need to consider each woman's needs individually rather than making blanket statements encouraging women to feel they must 'soldier on' or 'take the epidural' regardless of their personal circumstances, mindset, environment or support. In the 1920s, pain relief became a feminist issue, as women who were fighting for the vote on both sides of the Atlantic saw childbirth as another area in which women were lacking in agency and control. They were right but, again, we need to consider the type of birth from which they were interested in escaping – in this case, their choices were often either at home with a high chance of being attended by the doctor with his forceps, or, if you were working class, in dirty, poorly managed 'lying-in' hospitals. In the latter, death in childbirth was often at epidemic proportions due to 'childbed fever' – an infection caused solely by a lack of knowledge of the benefits of handwashing in doctors, who were often going between women and even to the morgue and back without considering deadly germs on their hands and instruments.[35]

If birth is horrific, it's a matter of human rights to want to absent yourself from it, and to the women of the early twentieth century, the ideal way of doing so seemed to present itself: Twilight Sleep. This method of pain relief, a mixture of morphine and the powerful narcotic and amnesiac scopolamine, placed women in a state of consciousness that meant they had no memory of giving birth at all. News travelled fast of a clinic in Germany that was offering these 'pain-free' births: 'The night of my confinement will always be a night dropped out of my life,'[36] said one woman who had experienced it, and she meant this in positive terms. Women began to demand Twilight Sleep as part of the new discourse about their autonomy, and the method spread across the USA, UK and Europe, with even Queen Elizabeth II using a version of the drug in the birth of her first three children in the late 1940s and 50s.

While the women who gave birth under Twilight Sleep remembered nothing, often to the extent that they felt no recognition for their own baby or were disbelieving that they had even given birth, the doctors and nurses witnessed a far less tranquil experience. Taken up as a way for women to gain more control in childbirth, the reality seemed very far away from this; women were placed in padded, crib-like beds, blindfolded, with cotton wool in their ears and their arms tied down or even straight-jacketed. Conscious, but entirely unaware of their own actions, the women under Twilight Sleep would thrash around and scream at full volume, often waking with feelings of disassociation and friction burns to their arms from fighting their restraint. This, along with side-effects such as horrifying flashbacks, increased birth complications and even death, caused the method to decline in popularity, but the use of scopolamine and the whole concept of 'knock 'em out, drag 'em out obstetrics' pervaded for sixty or more years of the twentieth century, interestingly, until another 'wave' of feminism came along to challenge the status quo.

As is so often the case, change started to happen when a man said what many, many women had already been saying and thinking, and suddenly the world took note. Grantly Dick-Read, in his 1942 book *Childbirth Without Fear*,[37] recalled a poor woman in Whitechapel some thirty years earlier who had given birth easily and without the chloroform he offered. 'It didn't hurt,' she had told him. 'It wasn't meant to, was it, doctor?' a phrase which stuck with him and inspired him to think about the effect of the mind on the body in labour, a concept that spread to the USA via another prominent male doctor, the Frenchman Fernand Lamaze. Dick-Read introduced the concept of the 'fear-tension-pain' cycle – we approach birth fearful and expecting pain, our bodies are tense, we therefore experience pain more deeply, and thus our pain is worse, and so on. For this pioneering thinking (which you can't help but assume was already fully on the radar of midwives and birth attendants since the dawn of time) Dick-Read has been named the 'father of natural childbirth'.

## Feminist awakenings

Dick-Read may have been the 'father,' but new ways of thinking had many 'mothers,' primarily birthing women themselves, who began to talk about the loss of dignity that came with pubic shaves, enemas, stirrups, restrained arms and hands, and obligatory narcotics. Bridget Baker, now a birth doula, worked in a UK maternity unit in 1964, as a nursery nurse. 'What I often saw and heard in the delivery room made me swear I would never give birth myself, but adopt instead. Women were often slapped, shouted at for making a noise, and told, "You helped to get it in there, now you help to get it out!"' There was a lack of available information for women, and what little advice that was given cast the person giving birth as entirely passive: 'In the delivery room, white with bright lights, you will be taken from the hospital trolley to the delivery table. The nurses will be standing by with the doctor and with their gentle help and encouragement, aided by the science they have studied so long, your baby will be born,'[38] read the *Sunday Express Baby Book* in 1950. In 1960, Queen Elizabeth opened a new building of the Royal College of Obstetricians and Gynaecologists with what she clearly felt was a glowing endorsement, 'You have given almost literal meaning to Wordsworth's assertion that, "Our birth is but a sleep and a forgetting".[39]

Not all women wanted to remain asleep, or as passengers and bystanders in their lives. Although the leading figures of the 1960's feminist movement did not have childbirth as a central concern, the new 'second wave' of feminism meant that thoughts and activism about women's rights in birth were still there in the zeitgeist. Inspired by her personal birth experiences, and by her reading of *Childbirth Without Fear*, in 1956 Prunella Briance set up the Natural Childbirth Association, which would go on to become the widely attended National Childbirth Trust or NCT. Its first stated aim was that 'women should be humanely treated during pregnancy and in labour, never hurried, bullied or ridiculed.'[40] In 1962 Sheila Kitzinger, already on the advisory board of the NCT, published her first book, *The Experience of Childbirth*,[41] which, when placed against the background of the times, still reads as revolutionary and extraordinary. Kitzinger's vision, inspired by her own anthropological studies, was of a 'Psychosexual Method,' in which birth was, 'part and parcel of the marriage and the love from the expression of which the baby owes his being'. Birth involved, 'one's relationship to life as a whole, the part one plays in the order of things,' and it was reasonable to expect, not 'suffering,' but 'joy': 'For far too many women pregnancy and birth is still something that happens to them rather than something they set out consciously and joyfully to do themselves,' she wrote.

Less than a decade after Kitzinger's book, Ina May Gaskin and her husband Stephen founded a commune known as 'The

Farm' in Tennessee.[42] There Gaskin started her midwifery centre, an out-of-hospital birthing community in which women were encouraged to birth naturally, in the presence of their partners and midwives, using active positions, and respecting the psycho-sexual energy of birth and the mind–body relationship. In 1979 she published *Spiritual Midwifery*, now a classic manual for home and natural birth. Filled with pictures of long-haired hippies and talk of 'yonis,' 'psychedelic rushes' and 'getting high' from the experience of labour, it was certainly not going to be on many obstetricians' recommended reading lists, and Gaskin's ideas may have stayed firmly at the fringe had she not published the birth stats from the farm in her 2003 *Guide to Childbirth*. In over two thousand births on The Farm between 1970 and 2000, their home birth rate was over 95 per cent, caesarean rate was 1.4 per cent, maternal mortality was zero and neonatal mortality was 0.39 per cent.* [43]

These extraordinary stats demanded Gaskin's ideas be taken seriously, but too late for the majority of women in the sixties and seventies who, in spite of Gaskin, Kitzinger, and the NCT challenging attitudes, could expect a heavily medicalised experience. The stand-ard obstetric approach became known as 'the active management of labour,'[44] with a focus on Friedman's Curve, developed in 1955 to chart a woman's dilation on a neat graph, and the standard way of judging the progression of labour even today. As midwife and

---

* Updated stats on The Farm website to 2010 confirm these results have continued. For comparison the USA home birth rate is 0.9 per cent (2017), caesarean rate 32 per cent (2018), neonatal mortality rate 0.58 per cent (2014), and maternal mortality rates are causing global concern.

researcher Dr Rachel Reed points out, this graph in itself dehumanises women, breaking them down into a set of parts and causing them to 'disappear' and be replaced by a diagram, rather than seeing them as a whole person.[45] This dehumanisation of birth, in which the clinicians look to charts, numbers, instruments and machines instead of the labouring woman, took hold in these decades and, because it has become so closely intertwined with people's view of safety, it is now extremely difficult to move away from. Twenty-first-century women themselves will assess whether or not they are in labour, or how fast things are progressing, not by how they 'feel,' but by what their contraction counting app is telling them. If birth practices somehow reflect the age in which we live, then it's fair to say that we live in an age which is at risk of losing human connection in favour of the electronic screen.

Screens are not all bad: the techno-medical model of birth has brought great improvements in safety. For 'high-risk' women, or in emergency situations such as post-partum haemorrhage, prematurity, placenta praevia, or truly 'stuck' babies, medical intervention can be life-saving. Unfortunately, healthy, 'low-risk' women are also getting this model of care, whether they need it or not. Improvements in birth outcomes in the twentieth century also owe a great deal to our improved overall health, better hygiene, and effective antibiotics, as much as the move to a hospital-based model. Sometimes I hear people or even professionals say, 'Don't forget women used to die in childbirth,' or 'Remember what birth is like in sub-saharan Africa' – implying that childbirth itself is inherently dangerous without medical management. But this is an over-simplification: women did not die in earlier centuries purely from the lack of modern obstetrics, but for different reasons, depending on the century, decade and location; from infection caused by the doctors themselves to obstructed labour due to conditions like rickets. They also died from conditions and in situations which modern medicine could undoubtedly have helped – this story is not either/or. And in low-income countries today, factors such as poor diet, health and hygiene, women giving birth at very young ages, and a lack of access to skilled care of any kind, also contribute to the danger of childbirth.[46] *And* women die in situations that access to modern obstetrics could undoubtedly save them from. Birth, in its safest form for healthy women, seems to require a combination: low-tech and midwife led, with easy access to medical back-up – but getting the balance right here seems to be difficult in our fear-based, litigation culture.

# Men's pleasure, men's convenience

What the modern medical package of care actually contains has changed from decade to decade, although at every point it has presented itself to women confidently and without apology. Rates of induction in the UK rose from around 15 per cent in the mid-1960s, to as high as 40 per cent in the mid-1970s[47] – a rate which – at 31.6 per cent in 2017–18[48] – we are now climbing towards again in the UK today. Birth moved decisively from home to hospital at this time, with UK home birth rates at around 5 per cent by the mid-1970s, where they have remained ever since. From the 1940s to the 1980s, routine episiotomy was commonplace, with as many as 60 per cent of women in the USA receiving this cut in the late 1970s.[49] Global rates remain high: one 2017 study found a rate of over 90 per cent in first-time mothers in Turkey.[50] Where there is a cut, there must be a stitch, and women who gave birth since the mid-twentieth century continue to report another symptom of health care misogyny, the so-called 'husband stitch'.

The idea that a doctor would put in an extra stitch or sew you tighter than necessary during suturing to make your vagina tighter for your (presumably male) partner is so shocking that many cannot even accept that it happens. Women report otherwise. Many say that while they were unsure if it actually physically happened to them, it was joked about in their presence either by professionals or partners, a scenario that is reflected in the 2017 short story 'The Husband Stitch' by Carmen Maria Machado,[51] which reignited the conversation about this practice.

> *They take the baby so that they may fix me where they cut. They give me something that makes me sleepy, delivered through a mask pressed gently to my mouth and nose. My husband jokes around with the doctor as he holds my hand.*
>
> *– How much to get that extra stitch? he asks. You offer that, right?*
>
> *– Please, I say to him. But it comes out slurred and twisted and possibly no more than a small moan. Neither man turns his head toward me.*
>
> *The doctor chuckles. You aren't the first*

This kind of scenario is unfortunately not restricted to fiction. Midwives report that the joke, 'Put in an extra one for me, doc,' is often made by partners, leaving health professionals feeling at a loss for words and awkward, and the woman feeling humiliated. Some health professionals will also joke about it, with one woman I spoke to from Cambridge, UK, telling me she was asked, 'Are we going for porn star then?,' during the stitching, while another, in Wales, was told, 'Don't worry, I am giving you a designer vagina.' Another woman, treated in Oxford, told me that her gynaecologist, while fixing a badly repaired episiotomy, joked that she could 'tighten me up a bit for my man while she was down there,' while another reported that after her birth in West London the midwife asked her husband to check her suturing to 'see if he was happy with it'.

In the USA, where routine episiotomy still happens in many hospitals,[52] the 'husband stitch' is more commonly reported – a spate of articles[53] in the wake of Machado's short story publication contained many first-hand accounts.[54] And in Hungary, a doula working there tells me one of her clients was told by her male obstetrician during suturing, 'From now on you will think of me whenever you are having sex with your husband.' In a recently reported case in Croatia, a woman given no anaesthesia and who was holding her newborn was told by the doctor, 'Stop shaking, hold still, I'm making you pretty for your husband.'[55] In Brazil, a doula tells me, 'It's very common. Most of the time it involves lots of jokes – "I will make you virgin again," "Your husband will like my work". Shockingly, many women even ask for it. The sexism is really inside the whole culture.' Whether the 'husband stitch' actually physically happens to a woman or if it is simply the subject of 'harmless banter,' the underlying objectification of women remains the same. Central to the concept of the stitch itself is the idea that women's bodies can be modified without consent to bring more pleasure to men, and this alone tells you everything you need to know about our current 'rape culture,' how violence against women is normalised and accepted in maternity as it is everywhere else, and why we need to start talking about #metoo in the birth room.

Whether or not you received an episiotomy or the offer of an extra stitch 'for daddy,' if you gave birth in the Western world any time since the 1950s, it's highly likely you were on your back. The story goes that it was Louis XIV of France who first popularised the idea of birth lying down in the seventeenth century, because he enjoyed watching his many mistresses deliver and this gave him a better view.[56] French doctor Francois Mauriceau is also credited with encouraging this position, which contradicts all the evidence for quicker, easier births and is rarely if ever observed in indigenous cultures or antiquity. The seventeenth-century Mauriceau, who is also believed to be one of the first to portray pregnancy as an illness or 'tumour of the belly,' wrote, 'The bed must be so made, that the woman being ready to be delivered, should lie on her back upon it, having her body in convenient figure.'[57] Convenient for care providers and observers, but positively unhelpful for women themselves, narrowing their pelvic outlet and meaning they are literally pushing their babies out 'uphill' and against gravity,[58] the position has nevertheless caught on, with around 60 per cent of UK women birthing on their backs according to a 2018 report, and 36 per cent with their feet in stirrups.[59] Over 90 per cent of US women lie on their backs for delivery,[60] and around 78 per cent of Australians.[61] In 1982, over 6,000 people marched in London at the Birthrights rally, responding to the lead obstetrician at the Royal Free Hospital who claimed that giving birth upright or on all fours was 'animalistic behaviour,' and made a labouring woman sign a disclaimer absolving the hospital of all responsibility if she refused to birth on her back.[62] The woman in question threw a jug of water over the staff. Led by Janet Balaskas, who pioneered the idea of active birth at this time, the march was joined by Sheila Kitzinger, Michel Odent, and newsreader Anna Ford, among others. 'It was almost like the need for a woman's body was becoming obsolete, once she'd carried the baby to term,' said Balaskas. 'It was like the plan was to get us into hospital, strap us into beds, pump us full of artificial hormones to get the process going, give us an epidural and if that didn't work then give us a Caesarean section.'

## Birth freedoms

While Balaskas was promoting active birth – a term that applies not only to the choice of mobile positions, but also encompasses women being 'active' rather than 'passive' in their choices – the epidural was taking hold as the 'go to' pain relief for labouring women, remaining the top choice to this day: around a third of UK women choose this option,[63] with much higher rates in other parts of the world, including over 60 per cent of women in the US[64] and as high as 80 per cent in France.[65] Epidural, which makes women numb from the waist down, usually results in very limited or no mobility, continuous electronic monitoring, an increased likelihood of instrumental delivery[66] (although this may be reduced by lower dose, more modern epidurals) and in the vast majority of cases, birth on your back.[67] Because of the lack of feeling, midwives or other attendants have to tell the woman when she is having a contraction, and when to 'push,' with some believing that the common practice of 'directed pushing' for all women, whether they have had anaesthesia or not, stems from epidural use. For some feminists, the epidural is the very epitome of freedom, releasing a woman from the destiny of her biology and 'Eve's curse'. 'It's interesting that no one cares very much about women doing anything "naturally" until it involves their being in excruciating pain,' wrote Jessi Klein in a 2016 article in *The New York Times*.[68] Others argue the complete opposite: it's female disempowerment at its finest, a 'devastating image' of 'female bondage' according to Adrienne Rich: 'Sheeted, supine, drugged, her wrists strapped down and her legs in stirrups, at the very moment when she is bringing new life into the world. This "freedom from pain," like "sexual liberation," places a woman physically at men's disposal, though still estranged from the potentialities of her own body.'[69]

Who is right? In our current polarised system, probably both. Women are now forced to choose between two models of care: the midwifery model and the medical model. Midwives, too, must choose which model they wish to conform to – do they become 'radical midwives,' working often at the edges of the system, independently from the NHS, attending mostly home births and supporting non-conformist choices such as HBAC (Home Birth After Caesarean), post-dates birth or vaginal breech, or do they become 'obstetric nurses,' unkindly referred to by some as 'med-wives,' conforming to the hospital-based system and keeping in line with its attendant policies and regulations? 'Opting out' of the obstetric-based system, if you are a birthing woman, is tough, and usually demands you have the privilege of both education and either the good family support and adequate housing that home birth demands, and/or the disposable income to hire an independent midwife (IM) – a choice that's become harder to come by in the past decade due to tighter regulations around insurance pushing many IMs out of practice.[70] If you do 'opt out,' you will probably also draw on the help of hypnobirthing, a birth pool, a doula, or all three, for pain relief. You might also arm yourself with knowledge about natural hormonal processes and make sure your birth room is uninterrupted, dark and warm. As you catch your baby with your own hands, you might feel that this 'freedom' empowers you and frees you from patriarchal control. If, on the other hand, you choose, or are forced for personal or economic reasons to choose, the medical model, you may find that your birth contains fewer of the elements that make pain manageable. You might find you are denied access to a birth pool. You might find you do not know your midwife. Your birth room may be brightly lit, sterile, and frequently interrupted. You may also find that your birth attendants are unable to break from protocol and allow your labour more time to unfold on its own terms. In this situation, as Jessi Klein argues, you might find yourself thinking, 'No one ever asks a man if he's having a "natural root canal." No one ever asks if a man is having a "natural vasectomy."' And she's right. If your birth presents itself as a medical procedure akin to dentistry or minor surgery on your nether regions, then yes, absolutely, the most empowered thing to do in that moment is get the epidural.

# A third way: relationship-based care

The history of birth is a history of power battles and, at the moment, the technocentric, dehumanised approach appears to be our chosen way forward. Our human attempts to control birth in the past 600 years or more have led us to this place where we perhaps feel we have almost completely won the battle against risk, but in which we might be wise to admit that something else has been lost. Sheila Kitzinger writes beautifully and extensively about the use of physical touch in birth and the postpartum period in other cultures, and of how nurturing, reassuring and comforting touch has been replaced in Western labours by manipulative, restraining and punitive touch.[71] Wires and machines so often take the place of human hands, and much of the touch from human hands themselves has become undignified and examining, rather than supportive. Her anthropological studies of birth are illuminating and show us just how much of the humanity and spirituality of the event have been swallowed up in the medical quest for safety. Maybe we have forgotten that we are the 'Doorway of the Mysterious Female' (Tao Te Ching), that our body is the 'House of Humanity' (Maori), and that when pregnant and labouring we might like to be celebrated, massaged and sung to, our birth room a fiesta of female company and support. In the postpartum period too, rather than being immediately urged to 'get back to normal' and 'get our bodies back,' perhaps we might like our curves and our softness to be rubbed with oils instead, while we are fed special foods and lullabied with verse about our life-giving achievements? Could this be, too, an aspect of being female, a lost dimension that, as feminists, we may wish to reclaim?

Instead, our tendency is to export our techno-medical approach to birth to indigenous cultures as the ultimate gift. Again, we don't need to see this in polarised terms: glorified natural birth in a remote hut vs. a stark and sterile hospital experience. The mother of birth anthropology (hooray, some fields have a mother!), Brigitte Jordan, advocated a two-way approach which she called 'fruitful accommodation,' where both indigenous cultures and Western medical practitioners listened to each other respectfully, acknowledging that there was something each could bring to and learn from the other. This could lead to growth on both sides, rather than a top-down imposition of the Western approach.[72] Similarly, qualities of midwifery that have been hard to quantify in the medical model, such as intuition[73] and emotional support,[74] have often been side-lined or even derided as unsafe. Jordan's 'fruitful accommodation' could be applied here too, encouraging a building of bridges between both approaches to childbirth, where neither is considered superior, but both learn from each other. As Professor Soo Downe writes, we need to start thinking in terms of 'both-and' not 'either/or': 'All those who want to improve maternity care, and outcomes for mother and baby, need to move to a "both-and" message. This is about both safety and positive experience; both mother and baby; both clinical and psychosocial outcomes; both short and longer-term benefits.'[75]

Both-and. Medical advances have brought so much that is good to childbirth, but if we wish to evolve a more humanised model of truly respectful care, we need to both hold on to those advances, and at the same time return to the roots of midwifery, the woman-to-woman care based on touch and connection, and the community-based support we have all but lost in recent decades. Delivering this kind of care demands a different model of maternity care to that which is currently available to most women, globally. All of the available evidence, coupled with the views of women themselves, suggests that a type of care known as 'continuity of carer' is the most likely to deliver on both safety and experience. Continuity of carer is usually midwife led and multi-disciplinary. It means knowing and having a relationship with your midwife that is built up during your pregnancy, so that you feel a human bond between you that incorporates and encourages two-way trust and respect. Working in this way has been shown dramatically to improve outcomes: in a Cochrane review based on 15 trials involving 17,674 women, those at low and higher risk who received continuity of care from a midwife they knew during the antenatal and intrapartum period (compared to women receiving medical-led or shared care) were 24 per cent less likely to experience preterm birth, 19 per cent less likely to lose their baby before 24 weeks' gestation, and 16 per cent less likely to lose their baby at any gestation.[76] Women were also more likely to have a vaginal birth, fewer interventions during birth, greater satisfaction with information, advice, explanation, venue of delivery, preparation for labour and birth, choice for pain relief, were more positive about their overall birth experience, and reported increased agency and sense of control, and less anxiety. Added to this, continuity of carer is also thought to be cost neutral.[77] For these reasons – and, equally importantly, because women overwhelmingly say they want it – the model has been recommended in the UK by the 2016 Maternity Review, known as Better Births,[78] who say the aim is, 'to ensure safe care based on a relationship of mutual trust and respect in line with the woman's decisions'. However, in the UK it's proving controversial to roll out nationally – in the main because being 'on call' for individual women who go into labour spontaneously and unpredictably is so very far from the shift work that many midwives are used to and around which NHS systems have been built for several decades. While some midwives love the continuity model, others say that it's impossible for them to deliver around family and other life commitments. Some even suggest that, in order to meet NHS targets, only pared-down versions of the model where women don't truly get the chance to build a rapport with their midwife will be offered. One anonymous midwife rather depressingly declared on Twitter that her trust intended to 'massage the figures' to meet continuity targets, and others report that their trusts are holding coffee mornings so that they can 'tick the box' to say that women have met their midwife before giving birth. Coffee mornings are undoubtedly a nice community event, but they are certainly not what is meant by 'continuity of carer,' and to try to meet targets in this way is disrespectful not just of the evidence that supports the continuity model, but of the women who would surely benefit from it in terms of both safety and experience. In the UK though, we are at least attempting to edge towards a continuity-based, midwife-led model – elsewhere in the world midwifery is often completely sidelined. In the USA, which has been named 'the most dangerous place to give birth in the developed world,'[79] almost all care is obstetrician led. And in Australia in 2018 one leading obstetrician accused midwives who use alternative therapies such as acupressure of practising 'dark arts,'[80] and the Australian Medical Association (AMA) have called for an investigation of the 'disturbing national trend'[81] of maternity care being midwife led. 'Obstetricians are the leaders,'[82] say the AMA, insisting that the evidence supports that obstetric-led care is safer, while consumer groups such as the Maternity Consumer Network say the opposite is true, and that furthermore, midwife-led continuity of carer is what women both desperately want and are struggling to access.[83]

Hundreds of years on from the Malleus Maleficarum, the birth power struggles and even the accusations of witchcraft continue. While overstretched maternity systems are part of the barrier to humanised, woman-centred care, a deeper problem is that the world remains suspicious of women's capabilities, and anxious not to let them have free rein in the act of bringing new life into the world. Can we move forward to a place where the power and control of birth is truly shared, passing into the hands of those who can best wield it in the woman's favour at any given moment? For this to happen, bridges will need to be built, and power that has been hogged for centuries by a patriarchal system will need to be restored to those to whom it belongs – birthing women. Likewise, broken trust will need to be repaired, allowing women to entrust their power back to the medical experts in times when their help is truly needed. The latter might be easier to achieve than the former: we've had decades of putting our faith in medical science for our births, and will probably, in that forgiving way that women often have, continue to do so. The real question is, as a culture, can we stop trying to take the power of birth away from women? Do we trust women to be the key decision makers about their bodies? Come to think of it, do we trust women?

# Chapter 4
# Loose Women

*Women, it seems, have an innate knowing of what
it means to burn ... and be burned. They know the
dangers in their bones. And it makes them wary.*

*Burning Woman,* Lucy Pearce[1]

Our freedom can perhaps best be measured by the way that
others react when we try to exercise it. Western women are
repeatedly told that they have 'choice in childbirth', but the stories
of 'loose women' – those who challenge, question, and generally try
to birth outside of certain norms and expectations – would suggest
otherwise. The idea that a woman must ultimately conform to
medical advice because this is always the safest route, and that she
must do this 'for the sake of the baby', is a hangover from the long
history of religious and patriarchal meddling in women's bodies
and lives, and continues to reach into every birth room.

# 'I am the expert here'

In 2012 I set up a network of free-to-attend antenatal discussion groups linked up by social media – The Positive Birth Movement (PBM).[2] At the groups, there is no teacher or expert, only a 'Facilitator', and instead women talk to and listen to each other, an approach sometimes called 'peer to peer' support. On PBM social media pages too, women are free to post questions about the choices they are facing, and gather differing views from an even wider variety of people than they would only have dreamt of having access to just a decade or so ago. What's not to like? you may ask, but on several occasions when I've described the structure of the PBM over the past few years, I've been asked, 'Is that *safe*?. Just a group of women, talking to other women, about their birth and their choices. Is that safe?'

The worry about PBM stems from concern that there is no 'expert' present, to guide the women and help them in their choices – disregarding of course that there are often researchers, obstetricians and midwives in the groups – because they can be female and even pregnant, too. But even if the groups and online conversations are entirely 'unsupervised', populated only with the 'unqualified' – do we really regard this to be *un*safe? If we are in a place where we have difficulty trusting women simply to have a conversation about birth with other women, then it's not really surprising that there is genuine anxiety in the birth room itself about who is the key decision maker. The ensuing power grapple – remember Kimberly's doctor saying, 'I am the expert here'[3] – is often about expertise, and about who 'knows best'. Polarised discussions position the 'floaty-dressed

149

woman' who believes in her body and trusts in Mother Nature, in direct opposition to the highly trained medical specialist. The conversation needs to shift away from tugs-of-war over who holds the expertise, and towards an understanding that, while the health care professionals may give fantastic advice, and may even have superior knowledge and experience, their role is to share this with the woman in their care, and after this, respect that she alone is the ultimate decision maker. Her body, her choice.

If you think this is already happening, think again. Unfortunately, we are still very much in a place where the edict is generally, 'Women are free to make any choices they wish about their births, as long as they are the right choices.' And whether or not they are the 'right' choices most often seems to be decided by someone other than the woman herself. If, when a woman gives birth, she feels free in her decisions, she may well be making choices that conform to certain expectations, and therefore not noticing any resistance. However, if she decides to make choices that do not meet with moral or cultural approval, she may find instead that her freedom is more restricted than she had anticipated.

## Policing birth choices

In 2012, when Melissa Thomas's son was seven days old, she received three visits in one day from social workers, operating under Section 47 of the Child Protection Act. On their third visit, at seven o'clock in the evening, they were accompanied by two uniformed police officers. Melissa, from Derby in the UK, was terrified that her two-year-old daughter and tiny newborn son were about to be taken into care. During their visits, including a 'welfare check' on their son the following day, Melissa and her husband were questioned in depth about their parenting choices, and their baby was weighed and measured without their consent, all on the premise that if they co-operated, this would soon be resolved. 'I felt empty, robbed of my free will,' says Melissa. 'I felt violated, persecuted – it was a witch hunt.' No charges were ever brought against Melissa, and the social services case was closed. And what had sparked this investigation? Melissa had voluntarily given birth at home, in her bath, with no midwife present. She was one of the many freebirthers who find themselves being reported to social services, an event that stays 'on file' forever, even if the concerns are decided to be unfounded. Sarah Holdway was reported by her health visitor for 'child trafficking' following her freebirth in Hull in 2016. Again, the case was closed and no action taken, but Sarah feels she is yet to get over it fully: 'To begin with I had nightmares and could not sleep, I was a wreck. Three years later I still sometimes have feelings of panic about it, for example if one of my children injures themselves, I think, will the doctors see my record and distrust me as a mother?' There are no exact figures on the numbers of UK women who freebirth, or which of those are reported to social services, but the Association for Improvements in Maternity Services (AIMS) say they have dealt with 'hundreds of cases' where birth choices have raised child protection concerns.[4]

How we choose to give birth is somehow seen to reflect our suitability as a mother, with the most points awarded to those who are compliant and unchallenging. Freebirth – a legal choice in most parts of the world – can be seen as a marker for reckless or unfit parents, and is closely monitored by both the press and social media. In the UK in 2015, J'Nel Metherell posted a birth announcement on her business Facebook page after a freebirth, only to have a midwife turn up on her doorstep the following morning to check on her baby. J'Nel believes she was being virtually 'watched'. A US-based group known as Exposing Freebirth takes this a step further, sending so-called 'Sock Puppets,' social media users with fake identities, into freebirth discussion groups, to watch their activity and some-times act on it – in November 2018, for example, they reported a labouring woman in Alaska resulting in two police officers turning up at her house. No action was taken and the woman transferred herself to hospital several hours later due to her own personal health concerns – but the Exposing Freebirth group nevertheless took the credit for 'successfully saving the life of the infant and its mother'.[5] 'These self-righteous bullies had nothing to do with my decision,' the mother concerned told me. In another high-profile case, a mother lost her baby at a freebirth in California, and 'sock puppets' who were part of the pro-freebirth group the Free Birth Society, screenshotted her story and shared it on social media. After labouring at home for three days, she had eventually transferred to hospital due to a severe bladder infection, where the doctors were unable to find a heartbeat. As she processed the loss of her baby, the woman was subjected to a torrent of online abuse and hate mail, calling her a 'Baby Killer'[6].

This kind of vigilante approach comes laced with a sense of entitlement and self-righteousness, and is sometimes, but not always, dished up with a side order of religion, a kind of logical progression from the Christian 'pro-life' argument. 'We know what is best for you and your body better than you do,' is, essentially, the attitude. But even if we try to debate the issue in a more level-headed, pro-choice way, the conversation can still get clouded by the very emotive and tragic reality of the loss of a baby, potentially – but not always – directly due to the mother's choice. Two questions are therefore important to consider. First of all, why is a mother who loses her baby at a freebirth – and sometimes this also extends to home birth attended by midwives – subjected to such moral scrutiny? We know that babies are tragically lost during hospital deliveries, in some cases, due to medical errors or negligence, in others, for reasons we are yet to explain or understand. In these tragic situations, the mother is never subjected to hatred or outrage. But when a baby is lost outside of the hospital setting, the need to find someone to expose, blame or punish seems to be universally urgent. Or to put it another way, we never ask, 'If this stillborn hospital baby had been born at home, could they have lived?'

If that argument still doesn't wash with you, and you feel that freebirth is, almost literally, taking freedom of choice a step too far, then let's consider the second question. If we decide that it's right to monitor or even police women's choice to birth unattended, because we believe that this will increase the chance of both mother and baby surviving, then what other birth choices do we feel should be banned, and what other interventions do we feel should be enforced? Maternity research is currently looking at whether interventions such as routine early induction could reduce stillbirth and other poor outcomes. If several trials confirm this to be the case, should women accept having their labours artificially started in hospital as the safest choice, and if they don't – if they choose to take a proven risk because they want a different kind of birth 'experience,' should we compel them to change their mind, either by hateful messages, social pressure, or even the law? And what other birth practices and interventions would we wish to see enforced, and on what basis? What kind of evidence would we want to see in order to compel or ban a certain action on the grounds of safety? Should all women birth in a medical setting? Should they all be induced? Should they all have caesareans? Perhaps we may eventually decide that the womb itself is too hostile an environment and that the baby will be safer if it is grown outside of the mother completely? A dystopian future begins to evolve if we allow our imaginations to progress too far down this route – a route which always starts with concerns for the safety of the baby over and above the experience, wishes, needs, hopes and desires of the mother.

Instead of getting our pants in a twist over women's irresponsible choices, it might actually be more interesting to ask a third question: why? Why do some women distrust hospitals and doctors? Why do they want to give birth without medical help? What positives are they gaining from this choice? When they carefully balance the risks of birthing outside the system, what are they putting on each side of the scales? It's so much easier to conceptualise these women as mad, hysterical, or just downright stupid than it is to actually tune in to them as rational humans and *listen*. If they *are* taking unnecessary risks with their own or their baby's life, what is driving this behaviour – their own personal failing as a mother or failings in the system? And what can the 'system' itself do to regain women's confidence, and build birth environments and models of care that they would not 'rather die' than experience?

These questions are not asked often enough. Meanwhile, we don't have to look into the world of fiction to find the dystopia that can occur when women's autonomy is ignored on a much greater scale than here in the UK – we need only travel as far as eastern Europe, where practices such as restraining women in labour, routine episiotomy, and the Kristeller manoeuvre – which involves applying huge pressure on the top of the bump during the 'pushing' stage – are all part of a maternity package that women have little choice but to accept. In September 2018 in the Lithuanian town of Siauliai, police were called to the hospital by obstetricians when a woman became 'aggressive' and 'overly emotional,' and refused to give birth on the 'birthing table'. According to reports, she was nearing the end of labour, wanted to stay on the floor, and did not wish to be examined. Initially, psychologists and psychiatrists were called, but when she still refused to agree, the police arrived, physically placed her on the table and held her by her arms as she gave birth to a healthy baby.[7] A report in the local paper showed no outrage, but instead, alongside an *actual image* of the woman being restrained, there was praise for the heroic actions of the police officers, and even a joke that perhaps the baby would grow up to be a policeman himself.[8]

In Croatia, MP Ivana Ninčević Lesandrić decided to speak out about her own experience of obstetric violence in October 2018, and her words before the parliament opened a floodgate of women's voices, with over 400 women sharing handwritten stories of their own experiences, including many who were not given adequate pain relief during obstetric interventions.[9] The women who have shared their stories have been widely condemned within the Balkans, and Lesandrić has been threatened with law suits by both the Minister for Health, and the hospital where she experienced mistreatment. The shocking treatment of labouring women in Croatia, and the fact that they are not permitted to question it, has its roots in (yup, you've guessed it!) patriarchy and religion, according to Zelijka Jelavic, a sociologist and lecturer at the Centre for Women's Studies in Zagreb. 'The starting point is the fact that the doctor is the one who knows and who has the power of decision,' she said. 'Added to this, I think that in our society, especially with the strong rise of the Catholic conservative right, the focus is put on the unborn child, not on the woman.'[10]

## Crazy choices

In the UK, while we may not be subjected to the Kristeller manoeuvre, the same underlying attitudes pervade, and rear their heads with gusto when women try to decline or opt out. Home birth is an option in UK care, but only if you meet certain 'low risk' criteria. Women who are 'high risk' but want to go ahead with their home birth anyway may be told, 'You are not allowed,' or 'It's against policy,' but a woman has the legal right to give birth where and how she wishes and midwives are obliged to respect her choices and have a duty of care to attend her. In spite of this, some hospital trusts in 2018 introduced worrying policies that suggested that midwives could decline to attend or even leave in the midst of a home birth if a woman refused their offer of an examination or a particular intervention – in other words, her care was conditional upon her compliance.[11] Women who are 'high risk' and therefore don't meet the strict criteria for home birth in the first place will almost always encounter barriers from their health care providers, ranging from mild discouragement to far more severe reactions, such as those experienced by Allie, a personal friend of mine who lives in a neighbouring Somerset village, and was referred to the psychiatrist by her obstetrician in 2015.

> *About 4 weeks before my second baby was due I*
> *was told that I couldn't have a home birth because I*
> *was high risk due to my age (41) my BMI, (32 at the*
> *beginning of the pregnancy) and having gestational*
> *diabetes (GD). It felt like the consultant spent the*
> *appointment telling me what would happen to me,*
> *'You will be induced at 38 weeks,' and so on, but when*
> *I disagreed and told him what we would prefer, he*
> *couldn't accept it. He spent the next 15 minutes talking/*
> *shouting directly at my husband and blanking both*
> *me and our independent midwife who had come with*
> *us, before storming out. All of his reasons were easy to*
> *counter with actual statistics but that just made him*
> *more angry. Afterwards we were all given an apology*
> *from the hospital midwife who had been sitting in*

*throughout for the way he treated us. The worst thing about it – with hindsight – was that because he was so busy trying to bully us into quietly going along with everything he wanted, he didn't look properly at the results of the scan that I had had just 30 minutes before. If he had, then he would have seen that our baby had stopped growing abruptly 3 weeks earlier, and so there was something potentially seriously wrong. We didn't know this until a few days later when I transferred over to another hospital because my blood pressure had risen and I wanted nothing to do with the original hospital. I was told there that we would have lost the baby within hours had the problem not been detected. In the meantime I received a phone call from the mental health team who explained they were calling as the consultant wanted to know if I was mentally fit to make decisions regarding my and my baby's care. I had a long chat with them on the phone anyway and they said they couldn't see any reason at all for them to say I was unfit and needed sectioning (which is what he wanted them to do) but we had to do it officially and make an appointment. My baby came before the meeting anyway, as he arrived 3 weeks early. At the time I was really angry and frustrated that the consultant thought it was OK to force me to do something to fit his own timetable or arbitrary guidelines, and was completely unwilling to listen to*

*either reason or statistics that didn't fit his view of*
*what should happen. He on the other hand felt that*
*spouting meaningless figures ('five per cent higher*
*risk than a younger woman'... etc) should mean that*
*I would do exactly what he demanded. He seemed*
*incapable of listening or taking on board anything that*
*we said to him. Three years on and I'm still annoyed*
*and frustrated that there are doctors like him out*
*there who can act in such a shameful manner but I'm*
*actually more angry at myself for not putting in a*
*formal complaint at the time. With all of the health*
*problems and hospital admissions that my baby had in*
*the first year it just went on the back burner and never*
*happened.*

'High risk' women like Allie meet the most resistance – as well as home birth, it can be equally difficult to birth in a midwife-led unit, and you may also find it impossible to access water birth. For all women, regardless of risk factors, declining scans or opting out of midwife appointments can cause problems: 'I wanted to opt out of antenatal care and my midwife phoned my husband to tell him that I'd missed appointments,' Sarah Thaw from Yorkshire told me. 'I thought this was a huge breach of my privacy and it made me feel like a child.' Antenatal appointments, ultrasound scans, blood tests, membrane sweeps, induction, vaginal exams, lying on the bed, monitoring, having your newborn weighed, vitamin K ... the list goes on. Part of the pregnancy package? If you're happy, fine.

Try and decline them, though, and you might start to get a bit more of a feel for just how free your choices actually are.

> *A rat in a maze is free to go anywhere, as long as it*
> *stays inside the maze.*
>
> Margaret Atwood, *The Handmaid's Tale*[12]

# Midwives with their hands tied

Another way in which women's choices can be policed and restricted is through the regulation and restriction of those who try to uphold or promote them. For women in the UK who wish to be supported in a birth outside of guidelines, an independent midwife – fully qualified, self-employed midwives who work for a private fee – is an option that is becoming increasingly difficult to come by. These midwives, who offer relationship-based, one-to-one care in a woman's own home, have a small army of supporters in the many women they've attended over the past thirty years or more, but this has not helped to secure their future. Ongoing wrangles over their insurance status have gradually chipped away at their existence, and although some still remain, in 2019 there are 32 registered with IMUK, a loss of around 50 since 2016, with many rural areas completely devoid of them.[13] Among those who do continue, there are concerns that persistent and ever-increasing scrutiny and regulation will eventually drive them out of existence. 'There are at least five IMs currently being investigated by the NMC,' one IM told me. 'Considering how few of us there are this is so disproportionate it would be funny if it wasn't for the fact that our careers and livelihoods are at stake if we do not comply.' With so few IMs left, this could be seen as a niche issue, but along with the independent midwives themselves, something greater is being lost – a model of midwifery centred around home birth, normality and woman-centred care, reliant on human interactions not machines – and if they cease to exist, this entire model risks dying with them. Independent midwives have the stats to show that the care they deliver is safe with one study finding no difference in outcomes between low-risk women with an IM vs. NHS care, and a straightforward vaginal birth rate of 77.9 per cent vs. 54.3 per cent in the NHS group. Babies born under the care of IMs in the study also had a significantly lower incidence of prematurity, low birth weight, and admission to the NICU.[14] IMUK say that they are determined to rebuild, albeit with higher fees – the cost of their escalating insurance must be passed on to women – making them inaccessible to most low-income families. It's hard not to get a sense of doom about the future of IMs, with some maternity safety campaigners portraying them as dangerous and irresponsible, and suggesting they should simply, 'take up jobs in the NHS'. This misses the point that if they are lost, there will be simply no alternative, other than freebirth, for UK women who feel unsupported in their choices by a protocol-heavy mainstream system.

In Australia, private practice midwives (PPMs), who work in a similar way to IMs, face similar battles. If you want to have a home birth in Australia, you may be out of luck, for the number of PPMs is in decline, mainly due to the absolute complexity of their regulation processes and to insurance demands that are difficult or impossible to meet. Since 2009, PPMs have had to have so-called 'collaborative relationships' with obstetricians, meaning that the choices of both midwives and the women in their care can effectively be vetoed by doctors.[15] 'This is a one-way collaboration,' Sydney-based PPM Jo Hunter told me. 'Midwives are mandated to collaborate, doctors can say "no, don't want to". This leaves PPMs powerless and only able to practise with the consent of a doctor. It's the ultimate patriarchal system and reinforces the medical domination of midwifery.' As a result of this and other regulation, women's choices have narrowed – for example birthing at home after caesarean, with twins, a breech baby, or past 41 weeks are all against guidelines – and those who have tried to continue to uphold a model of maternity care based around a woman's freedom to make her own choices have risked persecution.[16] Says Jo Hunter, 'PPMs are getting reported when they support women who choose care outside recommended guidelines. I don't think anyone would find a PPM willing to take on known twins or known breech at home, it's career suicide.'

Midwives can often be placed in the firing line, and it seems that usually they are the midwives who promote models of care built entirely on women's choices, rights and bodily autonomy. Maureen Collins works for One to One Midwives, a service that since 2010 has offered a caseloading midwifery model – in which women are cared for by a midwife they know – in the north-west of England and Essex. This service is free to women under the NHS, and in the past five years (to 2018), they have collected data on their work with over 8,000 women. This shows their normal birth rate to be 97 per cent at home births and 76 per cent at home and hospital, compared with the national figure of 59.4 per cent. Their stillbirth rate is almost half the UK number at 2.3 per 1,000, their neonatal death rate is 4 times lower than the national figure, and their neonatal admission rate at term is 8 times lower.[17] 'Our philosophy is to support women in their human right to birth where and how they wish, but most of the time, I find myself trying to protect the organisation from criticism and at worst, being closed down,' Maureen told me. 'The biggest issue is the current system does not trust women to make an informed choice, we are seen as mavericks outside of that, because our whole model is based on reproductive autonomy.' Women who wish to go against guidelines have their sanity questioned: 'I am constantly asked, "Does she have capacity?,"' Maureen tells me. Midwives from One to One are often referred to the NMC (their regulatory body). 'Mostly it comes to nothing but the pressure has caused one or two of them to leave the profession. There is excessive scrutiny, and no attention paid to our outcomes. If people cared about outcomes, our service would be rolled out across the country. Instead we are constantly under threat.'

Maureen is right to be concerned – precedents have been set for the shut-down of woman-centred models that are brave enough to challenge the status quo. From 1997 to 2009 the Albany Midwifery Practice[18] was part of the King's College Hospital Trust in south-east London, providing care to just over 2,500 women during that time, in an area with high levels of socio-economic disadvantage. Fifty-seven per cent of women served by the Albany were from black, Asian or minority ethnic (BAME) communities, one-third were single mothers and 11.4 per cent identified themselves as both single and unsupported. The Albany offered true continuity, with over 95 per cent of women in their care being attended in labour by either their primary or secondary midwife. They created a community-based model, with antenatal and postnatal groups for women in the area, and an encouragement of women to decide on home or hospital birth as late as they liked in their pregnancy, or even during labour. They took on both high- and low-risk women. And their stats were extraordinary, in particular when compared with UK-wide stats from the same period (in brackets)[19]: 6.5 per cent induction rate (25 per cent), 16 per cent caesarean (26.2 per cent), 79.8 per cent spontaneous vaginal birth (60.9 per cent), and 43.5 per cent home birth (2.3 per cent). Epidural rates were low at just under 10 per cent and around a third of women used water immersion in labour. Also notably low were their rates of perineal damage with two-thirds of Albany women who birthed vaginally having no tears at all, only 0.7 per cent having third-degree tears, and none having fourth-degree tearing. For comparison, RCOG state that around 90 per cent of women will tear during birth, with third- and fourth-degree tears currently causing concern at around 6 per cent and rising.[20]

In spite of being not only highly valued by the local community in Peckham, but also held up as an example of both ground-breaking and outstanding midwifery practice internationally, the Albany was closed suddenly and without any consultation by the King's College Trust in 2009, due to safety concerns. There was widespread protest at the closure, including a 'Reclaiming Birth' rally in 2010 attended by over 2,000 people,[21] but to no avail. Their perinatal mortality rate was around half that of the London borough of Southwark where they were based, and their practice has been found by independent researchers to be beyond exemplary,[22] but in spite of this the Albany has never been reinstated. Nor have the Albany ever received any kind of apology from the Trust, who for many years had a statement on their website claiming that their investigation found, 'serious shortcomings in terms of non-compliance with Trust policies and risk management procedures'.[23]

Becky Reed, one of the small team of Albany midwives, told me, 'It seemed at the time, and seems now, that there were forces at work wanting to discredit a midwifery care model that put women's choice at the heart of its philosophy, inevitably leading to a huge increase in home birth. I think for some obstetricians and "risk managers" this caused a massive amount of discomfort, and led to a desire to wipe the Albany (with its incredibly positive outcomes) off the map.' Reed was initially suspended at the time of the closure, and then referred to the NMC. After a three-and-a-half-year investigation that Reed referred to as a 'witch hunt,' the case against her was dismissed when the NMC failed to offer any evidence, and, again, no apology has ever been made for these actions.[24] Reed is by no means alone in her identity as a woman-centred midwife who has been singled out, tried, persecuted or even metaphorically burned. Agnes Gereb, an obstetric doctor turned midwife, has worked tirelessly to humanise birth in her native Hungary. As early as the 1970s she was suspended from practice for smuggling fathers into the delivery room, who were at the time forbidden. 'The freedom of a country can be measured by the freedom of birth,' she said, which somehow neatly sums up both how much one determined woman can do for the freedom of birthing women internationally, and the toll this can take on her personal liberty: Gereb has changed the face of birth at great personal expense. Charged with attending home births including two at which a baby died – the only baby deaths in her twenty-year home birth practice – Gereb has endured decades of persecution including trials, imprisonment, and years of house arrest.[25] She has appeared in court with her legs shackled and her arms handcuffed. In early 2018 she received a two-year prison sentence, but was then granted clemency by the Hungarian president after immense international pressure.[26] Supporters worldwide recognised the injustice of her situation and the great contribution she has made to human rights in childbirth, not least due to her involvement in the landmark case in the European Court of Human Rights, Ternovsky vs. Hungary, which established a woman's right to give birth where and how she chooses.[27] Gereb has consistently upheld the right of a woman to autonomy and choice, and she has lost decades of her personal freedom as a result.

To explore the cases of other midwives who have faced persecution would possibly take another book. From Ireland to Australia to the Netherlands to the USA and Brazil, the sight of a midwife in the dock or even in handcuffs is not as obsolete as you might assume in the twenty-first century. The high-profile cases that make the news are just the tip of the iceberg though, and what lies beneath is a profession on edge, conflicted between the traditional role of 'mid-wife' which literally translates as 'with woman,' and a strong driving force in many maternity units that insists on policies and protocols that focus on the survival of mother and baby but often ignore the experience of childbirth as a meaningful and spiritual rite of passage. Again we see polarisation, between those subversive midwives who may jokingly refer to themselves as a 'midwitch' and others who conform to the medicalised system and become 'medwives' or 'obstetric nurses'. Non-conformists may work outside the system as independent midwives or doulas, or stay within it and try to make a stand for women, for example by promoting more woman-centred models of care, or even by small acts of rebellion such as recording the progress of a woman's dilation inaccurately so that she is 'allowed' more time before policy dictates intervention is necessary. Those who like to work outside of guidelines or think outside the box may face criticism – obstetrician Niamh McCabe, who supports women wishing to birth vaginally after caesarean in Ireland, told me, 'Sadly, I have experienced many negative effects of supporting women's choice. I am made to feel like a maverick, I get repeated comments about how "brave" (they mean "bonkers") I'm being to support women who dare to opt for care which is not the standard, I have to go on call for women myself when colleagues will not support them.' Many others who try to make changes experience bullying. Amanda Burleigh, an award-winning midwife and a pioneering voice in the UK and globally against the practice of immediate cord clamping,[28] has left the profession due to what she describes as '15 years of bullying and intimidation'. 'In raising my head above the parapet in order to challenge and change routine non-evidence-based practice, I was forced from a job I loved,' she told me. 'Rather than protecting staff, parents and babies, the system seems geared towards brushing accountability and informed choice under the carpet. What sort of profession silences their most passionate staff? The answer is a profession in danger.'

# THE PERFECT BIRTH ENVIRONMENT

Women are mammals. Ask any self-respecting cat where they want to give birth, and they will tell you, in a warm, cosy, dark and undisturbed place. Ask any zoo keeper how they help their labouring pandas and they will tell you, by making them a warm, cosy, dark and undisturbed place. But in this world that understands mammalian needs so well, we seem collectively baffled as to why women's labours stall or 'fail to progress' when they turn up at brightly lit, busy obstetric units. Just like all other mammals, human birth is reliant on the interplay of hormones, primarily oxytocin, which, you've guessed it, likes warm, cosy, dark and undisturbed places. The fact that this knowledge is not built into the design of every maternity unit is detrimental to women on a huge scale and should top the agenda of anyone who wants to make birth a better and safer experience.

In the meantime, what can you do to create an environment that supports your female physiology?

### Have a home birth or birth centre birth

Home is where most of us feel safest, and the next best option is a birth centre or midwife-led unit, where more focus is usually given to creating a dimly lit, woman-centred environment. Access to home birth or MLU may vary depending on where you live in the world and your own personal circumstances. A large-scale study in the UK called the Birthplace study has found that birth at home or in a birth centre is safer for the mother in terms of avoiding major medical interventions. One of the elements that makes home birth so safe is access to good medical back-up, so you need to consider your access to obstetric help – for example, time and distance to the hospital – when making this choice.

## Know your three brains

Giving birth is primal. When choosing where you want to have your baby, you need to realise that, in labour, the part of your brain that is responding to your surroundings will be your deeper, limbic brain, not your rational, intellectual neocortex. (The third part of your brain, the cerebellum or reptile part, is less relevant.) So choosing your place of birth is not about asking, 'Where do I *think* is safest?' but 'Where do I *feel* safest?'

## Get the basics on the love hormone

Understand the ins and outs of the hormone oxytocin, the main player in the birth process. Some call oxytocin the love hormone, as it is involved in falling in love, sex, orgasm, birth, bonding and breastfeeding, but it's also known as the 'shy hormone' as it likes to be . . . warm, cosy, dark and undisturbed. If you think of a typical 'romantic' environment – candles, soft light, favourite music, a log fire and absolutely no interruptions, you are not far off the ideal birth room. The kind of place you would like to have really loving sex in, basically.

## Protect your birth space

Wherever you birth, but especially if it's away from home, make sure you keep interruptions during labour to a minimum. Nervous partners might like the TV on or to chat away to you throughout, but their needs must be put aside and you must be given the chance to 'get in the zone' and, once in that zone, not be constantly brought back out of it. Birth partners, dads or doulas, can be tasked with protecting the birth space, making sure curtains stay drawn, lights stay off and visitors keep away.

## Build a nest

Use sheets or blankets, cushions, yoga mats and pillows to make a place to retreat. This could be in your house or in the corner of your hospital room. Use ear plugs or an eye mask to block out light and audio/visual stimulation. Alternatively wear headphones and listen to a playlist. Shut out the world and focus.

## Choose love

You can up your oxytocin production by focusing on love. Have photos of people or places you love or happy times in your life near you in your birth space. Connect with your baby and think about the love you already have for them and how this will grow once they are born. Be loving with your partner, and if you feel like it, smooch and 'make out,' or if you are alone, masturbate – orgasms, kissing and nipple stimulation can up your levels of the love hormone you need to birth and are a great thing to try if your labour stalls.

## Taboo topics

In recent years, I've personally observed not just the policing of women and professionals' behaviour in the birth room, but also the policing of thoughts and opinions around birth itself. Speaking regularly at birth conferences around the UK and globally, as I do, I can tell you from personal experience that there is a great deal of anxiety, particularly among midwives, about the language used in relation to 'normal,' 'natural' or 'physiological' birth. The 'promotion of normal birth' is part of the international definition of the midwife[29] – to put it in very basic terms midwives' entire outlook is rooted in how female physiology 'works' and how to help this happen – this is their passion. However, in the summer of 2017, it was widely reported in the UK press that the Royal College of Midwives had suddenly dropped the term 'normal birth'.[30] A deluge of news articles appeared, many of which also referred to the 2015 Morecambe Bay Enquiry, an investigation into a series of tragic deaths of mothers and babies at the Furness General Hospital.[31] The enquiry at Morecambe Bay found that 'a series of failures at almost every level' were responsible, but many media reports attached 100 per cent of the blame to the so-called 'musketeer midwives,' a group who were determined to, in the words of the report, 'pursue normal childbirth at any cost'.

It seemed like the RCM were dropping not just the term, but the whole concept of 'normal birth,' perhaps even in response to Morecambe Bay. But in fact, the RCM had ended their 'Campaign for Normal Birth' in 2014, and while the news coverage therefore seemed to be a non-story, this didn't stop the then Health Secretary

Jeremy Hunt from tweeting about it, claiming the RCM terminology change would 'help the government plan to halve neonatal deaths and injuries'.[32] While there are valid arguments to be had about the term 'normal birth,' which some women may experience as a value judgement, the point here is deeper than semantics – it's about a really strong, quite successful, and highly inaccurate attempt to associate 'normal' or 'natural' birth with danger and death.[33] Somehow, this twist on the actual facts of the story was successful, and many people's 'take home' point from the press coverage was simply '*midwives are not allowed to talk about normal birth any more because it's dangerous*'.

This is a fairly accurate summary. Two of the UK's leading midwives have since been 'exposed' in the press for giving their views on natural childbirth. In November 2017 Sheena Byrom OBE was reported by the *Daily Mail* to be 'giving talks that allowed midwives to be exposed to pro-natural birth messages,'[34] while in March 2018, former RCM president Caroline Flint was outed in *The Times* for having said that doctors were 'hopeless at childbirth' and that their wages might be better spent on employing more midwives.[35] Whether or not Flint's comments were helpful or accurate, it's rather chilling to consider that she made them while *in the audience* at a midwifery event. They may have been off the cuff, ill considered or even intended in jest, but nevertheless they were recorded and widely reported to her detriment. There's certainly a feeling at midwifery and birth events at the moment that the walls have ears, and words need to be watched.

It's important to remember, of course, that what may seem like 'surveillance' or 'persecution' to some is simply 'regulation' to others. Those who believe that maternity safety will only be achieved by technocracy and the absolute dominance of obstetrics will certainly not feel that there is anything wrong with pulling into line those women and midwives who misguidedly think there is a value to 'hands off,' 'physiological' or even 'normal' birth. This would not be a feminist issue if the move to medicalise childbirth further were indeed the only way to make it safer, or if women did not mind about high-intervention experiences, or similarly if women collectively felt indifferent to the idea of an empowering, uplifting birth experience – but this is not the case. The question of what makes birth safe and how we might make it safer, we will come to in the next chapter, but, for now, let's talk about sex.

## Yes! Sex!

The idea that birth and sex are connected sometimes comes as a shock to people. We're taught to think about the two bodily acts in very different ways. Imagine if I asked you to brainstorm the words you associate with each of the two. Sex? You might give me: fun, loving, erotic, pleasurable, exciting, orgasmic. Childbirth? Most people would say: painful, bloody, gory, agony, horrific, scary. You can see why the two activities are not very often associated! But of course they are – deeply associated. Sex and childbirth in fact have quite a lot in common. Hopefully some of the basics go without saying: sex is how a baby gets in, and childbirth is how that same baby gets out.

In some ways, it could be said that childbirth is the true 'climax' of sex – it certainly could be seen as the final moments of a story, and an ending as well as a beginning of one of life's many cycles. Sex and birth involve the same parts of the female body, and the same 'love hormone,' oxytocin, is produced during orgasm and is essential for labour, too. For some women, this crossover is experienced physically: a 2016 survey of 2,200 mums by Positive Birth Movement and Channel Mum found that 6 per cent reported having orgasmic births[36] – at 1 in 20, that figure is perhaps surprisingly high.

A woman who is labouring freely and uninterrupted, choosing her own positions, following her instincts and spiralling deep into that place some refer to as 'the zone' or 'labourland,' will not look dissimilar to a woman in the throes of sexual pleasure. She may rock on all fours and moan, with her mouth open and her eyes closed. 'I often find myself thinking, "This is a bit like a porn film," I'm not sure I should even be here!' one midwife told me. Shalome Stone from Melbourne, Australia, had an orgasmic birth in 2013. Inspired by viewing a film of ecstatic birth online, she decided that, if this was possible for the woman in the film, it was possible for her, too. 'I thought, yes please, I'll have what she's having,' she told me.

*It was a fast and furious birth, just two and a half hours from start to finish. It was intense, and I remember thinking, 'Oh wow, this is either about to get really painful, or I can dig deeper and make it amazing.'*

*I dug deeper and let go. And I mean, I really let go. I
was on fire – every fibre of my being was engaged and
pulsing. Another wave started and I focused on the
build-up, breathing deep, surrendering to the intensity,
riding, riding, riding and then … throwing my head
back, moaning out loud. It was the most incredible
rush, more sensual than sexual. I have never felt more
feminine, more goddess-like, more womanly, than in
that moment. That birth taught me the magic and
beauty that can happen when a woman is able to birth
in a safe, familiar place, with her loved ones, with a
dedicated midwifery team, and with the self-belief that
she is capable of greatness.*

The connections between birth and sex go beyond the physical.
Female sexuality has a long history of being repressed. In the past,
women have been made to 'lie back and think of England,' and
have been persuaded to think of sex as something that must be
endured, rather than enjoyed. In the same way, women continue
to be placed on their backs in childbirth and encouraged to be
passive and patient until it is over. Sheila Kitzinger, who felt that
our Western society infantilised labouring women and 'de-sexed'
them, made the point that we tend to view the climax of birth
through a lens of male rather than female sexuality. 'Instead of the
wave-like rhythms of female orgasm, bearing down is treated like
one long ejaculation: stiffen, hold, force through, shoot!' she wrote.
'Any sexual feelings are completely eradicated.'[37]

In both birth and sex, we still have a poor understanding of women's bodies, how they are built, what they need, and how they work best. In a world where many of us still don't know our vagina from our vulva, we struggle to teach our daughters about their basic anatomy, because we have never learned it ourselves. The debate is ongoing about what girls should be told in class about the anatomy and function of the clitoris[38] (much of which has only recently begun to be understood).[39] Menstruation continues to be taught as a rather unpleasant bodily function and is never marvelled at or welcomed, let alone celebrated as a female rite of passage. We leave topics like female masturbation and the female orgasm out of sex-ed completely, and in a similar way there is anxiety around teaching young people about childbirth as a powerful and positive experience. The myth persists that if we are honest with girls about the wonders of their bodies we may somehow encourage them into engaging with their physicality and sexuality in a way that remains culturally unacceptable – that they may even become 'loose women'.

*She had blood coming out of her eyes. Or blood coming out of her wherever.*

Donald Trump on Fox News's Megyn Kelly[40]

Why do we still find loud, raucous, visceral, intuitive, strong, lusty, angry, leaky, opinionated, independent women difficult to accept? These 'loose women' are the ones who have broken free, we cannot contain them, they are wild and unrestrained. They are the ones who will not 'take it lying down,' they want to 'stand on their own two feet,' or be 'on top,' they are the movers, shakers and troublemakers. In the bedroom and in the birth room, we have historically tried to keep these women still, quiet and restrained. The 'good' woman continues to be the one who complies and does not cause trouble. She will lie still, and passive, and let it be done. And, as we have seen in this chapter, those who will not comply can no longer be literally burned, so our patriarchal culture finds other ways of either silencing them, or making an example of them so that others are silenced. We threaten their livelihoods and their reputations, call them bad mothers and warn that we may take away their children. We suggest they are mad, put them in the dock, expose them in the media or even take away their freedom.

Just as women were once told, 'sex is for procreation and nothing more,' they are now told, 'childbirth is for procreation and nothing more'. In either act, what matters is the production of a healthy baby, and the woman is merely the means to that end. The experience of childbirth is dismissed as meaningless and unimport-ant to a woman's body, heart or soul, just as the experience of sex used to be. And why? What is to be gained by these oppressions? The reasons are the exact same reasons whether it's birth or sex: because in these places can be found both power and pleasure. To uphold the patriarchy, women must be cut off from any experience that connects them to a sense of power or strength, and the idea that they and their bodies are weak and inferior must be reinforced.[41] They must believe that they cannot give birth without help, and this in turn supports capitalism – natural birth doesn't cost very much – and helps keep men 'on top'. Women who have empowered births often say that it changed their life, and that they would 'never again be afraid of anything'. To the patriarchy, this is potentially dangerous. The medicalisation of childbirth has accelerated in recent years, in direct correlation to the increase in women's voices and power in other areas: one wonders if this is a coincidence. Or is childbirth the last frontier, both a crucible of our powerful potential as female humans, and, at the same time, our Achilles heel, an overlooked gap in our armour?

A woman in labour, upright, roaring, delivering her own baby and catching it with her own hands challenges everything people assume to be true about childbirth, and is the antithesis of the sanitised, objectified woman, covered by drapes, silenced by drugs or even devoid of pubic hair. This roaring, birthing woman is real, naked, shameless, capable, useful, active, empowered. And, culturally, we find this an awkward energy to be around – it is loud, and raw, and sexual. As one old-school midwife put it to a doula friend of mine, 'It's *unseemly* – wouldn't she feel more comfortable with an epidural?' In the bedroom and the birth room, there persists a fear of the loose woman and her potential. 'Home birth, natural birth . . . these are acts of civil disobedience,' Professor of Midwifery Hannah Dahlen said to me. 'The hand that rocks the cradle does rule the world. And if that hand is powerful then the children that step from that cradle are centred and certain and much harder to manipulate with fear, which is after all the main tool of capitalism and the number one strategy of men in power.'

Fear. Fear is key to oppression and control, and in the twenty-first-century birth room, it's big, and it's everywhere. We make our choices and we hope they are free and informed choices, but, much of the time, they are informed by one thing, and one thing only – fear. Fear is at the root of all birth power struggles; it is there when we challenge, and it is there when we conform. Pregnant women are often told to counter the fear with self-belief, with birth 'affirmations' like, 'She believed she could, so she did,' 'Trust in your body,' and, 'You were made to do this'. But perhaps the enemy of fear is not confidence, but information; when we can name Rumpelstiltskin, he loses his power over us. Birth will never be straightforward in every case – we need modern obstetrics just as much as we need cancer drugs and anaesthetics. But as women and as feminists, with a long history of having our choices policed and our bodies controlled, we need to ask ourselves this: *how many of us who are getting help from obstetrics actually need it?* This is the big question, and the answer we collectively reach will decide the future of childbirth. This, in turn, impacts on the lifelong physical and psychological health of women and babies, and by extension their families, making it a question of fundamental importance to humanity.

# Chapter 5
# Women's Bodies: Unfit for Purpose?

*Her wings are cut and then she is blamed for not knowing how to fly.*

Simone de Beauvoir, *The Second Sex*[1]

I can clearly remember the moment when I first discovered I was pregnant. I was alone in the house, and having peed on the testing stick, I waited, feeling frozen in time, as though precariously balanced on a tipping point. Without realising it, pregnancy test manufacturers have created something truly poetic – women in bathrooms and cubicles everywhere now sit and stare as a pale line slowly appears, getting darker . . . and more believable . . . until there is no doubt left . . . and the line between a past life and a future life has been both literally and metaphorically drawn. Suddenly everything that has gone before that moment seems to belong to an entirely different era, an entirely different human even.

After the positive test, the new, pregnant me stood in front of the bathroom mirror and stared at my reflection. I didn't look any different. But I was. My first thoughts, though, did not revolve around nursery paint colours, or giggling curly-locked little children running towards me in corn fields. Even though I wanted this baby and had planned to get pregnant, my first thoughts were mainly along the lines of 'OMG there's a baby in there', swiftly followed by 'OMFG it's got to get out.' Even in those first moments of realising my pregnancy, my overriding emotion, apart from incredulity and shock, was *fear*.

I looked at my reflection, at my slender frame and at my narrow hips. I thought about the taut skin of my midriff. I thought about my vagina and how small it was. And then I thought about watermelons, bowling balls, wrecking balls, pineapples coming out of nostrils, and biblical camels trying to squeeze, against all hope, through the eyes of biblical needles. In short, I thought about everything that was going to have to stretch and expand in a way that didn't seem humanly possible.

# The broken chain of wisdom

I had never been anywhere near a birth, nor had I held or even touched a newborn baby. Like many modern women, my only frame of reference for birth was the diabolical school video, the usual overheard snippets between family members, and pub jokes about the horrors of childbirth. Birth had moved out of the community and into the hospital long before I was born, meaning that my mother, like me, had had a similar lack of exposure to childbirth; women simply went to the hospital pregnant and came back with a baby, and what happened in between remained a mystery. I call this state of affairs 'the broken chain of wisdom' – that matriarchal lineage through which knowledge, experience and deep understanding is passed, has slowly but surely lost many of its links and connections. This also applies to breastfeeding – we no longer see it around us, and our first experience of it may well be when we are trying to do it ourselves.

In any void, something is bound to stir into life. The current gaps in women's wisdom about birth are dark and fertile places, where the seeds of fear can very quickly germinate. Researchers currently estimate that around 14 per cent of women are affected by tokophobia[2] – the pathological fear of going into labour and giving birth. The exact numbers of women who are either genuinely tokophobic or affected by a lower-level state of fear and anxiety about childbirth are difficult to measure, but you only have to talk to women of childbearing age to discover just how common it is to find birth scary, off-putting, disgusting, horrifying or terrifying. And, of course, young women become midwives and obstetricians as well as mothers, so fear of birth is brought to the table by professionals, too. Studies have found that between a quarter[3] and a third[4] of female obstetricians would personally choose a caesarean birth, with many citing the trauma they have seen in their working life as the key motivating factor. Research in Australia has found that not only are a high proportion of midwives fearful of birth or traumatised by their personal or professional experiences, but that this has a direct impact on their practice – highly fearful midwives are less confident in the support they give to pregnant and birthing women.[5]

If you are pregnant, and reading this book, you probably find yourself somewhere on this spectrum of fear, from the mildly anxious to gripped by a terror so strong that you may have resisted having children for a long time and may now wish there was another way out of pregnancy than birth itself for you. Those whose fear is intense enough to receive a diagnosis of tokophobia are split into two categories – 'primary tokophobia' in those women who have never been pregnant or who are in their first pregnancy, and 'secondary tokophobia', in those who have had a previous traumatic birth and are basing their fear on bitter experience. Wherever women are on the spectrum of fear, the fears they list have much in common, it is generally only the intensity that varies. Commonly cited are: 'losing control', 'pain that I can't handle', 'tearing and damage to my body', or 'something going wrong'. Some fear the great responsibility for another life that pregnancy and labour bring, and this may be exacerbated by the current intense pressure on women to be a textbook 'perfect mother'. Many, as I was, are afraid of needles, scalpels and other interventions that may happen to them as part and parcel of having their baby. And just like me when I stood in front of the mirror, the basic question that underpins many women's fears is simply, 'How is it going to get out?' It just doesn't seem possible.

## Too much of a stretch?

For all of us, then, this question of 'are women's bodies fit for purpose – do they "work"?' is not just feminist theory, it's a vital, practical and very real concern. If you're already a mother, and were one of the majority of women for whom the experience was not straightforward, you may want to know if what happened to you that day was the only possible way things could have gone. If you haven't had a baby yet, you might want to know if there's any chance that you can get that camel through the eye of that needle, or if you might as well give up now and hand yourself over to the obstetricians. And as women, whether we are mothers, mothers-to-be, or even if we don't ever plan to reproduce, we need to consider the question for the sake of our friends, sisters and daughters. Does birth work, or is the female body simply a design fault?

For all my adult life I can remember being told that human birth is difficult because we have evolved to walk upright. I'm not sure the explanation ever got much deeper than that, and, often, it still doesn't. In the frequent Twitter debates that rage about the sky-rocketing levels of birth intervention, someone often will tell me, 'It's because we used to be apes. Now we walk upright and have intelligent babies with big heads. That's why childbirth doesn't work quite right without medical help.' This isn't just twitterings, though, it's 'proper science'. Known as the 'obstetric dilemma', the theory is that we have had to reach an evolutionary compromise in order to continue to birth our young. Female humans have had to develop pelvises just wide enough to accommodate larger-brained babies, but just narrow enough to allow them to walk on two legs. This makes human birth more difficult than that of other mammals and means that babies need to be born as early as possible, rendering them dependent for longer than their primate counterparts. And the obstetric dilemma has implications beyond childbirth – the larger female pelvis means that women are less physically able than men – or so the theory goes.

The obstetric dilemma may be oft-quoted, but two things are important to bear in mind. First and foremost, it's only a hypothesis – put forward in 1960 by the American anthropologist Sherwood Washburn – and secondly, it has been challenged and discredited, most notably by Rhode Island anthropology professor Holly Dunsworth. In 2007, she became curious about how a theory that suggested women were biologically 'compromised' in some way could be so widely accepted. She noted that women had quite wide variety in the size and shape of their birth canal, and yet all seemed to have no problems in walking. Dunsworth looked to Harvard researcher, Anna Warrener, who tested the notion that women's wider hips made them less efficient at locomotion – and found it to be incorrect. Men and women are both equally efficient at walking and running.[6]

Warrener's research was unable to demonstrate female inefficiency – and the theory that being a woman is a kind of physical disability in itself thankfully seems to have been debunked – at least as far as walking and running are concerned. But what about birth? Are we compromised here in some way? Dunsworth thinks not.[7] Although she acknowledges that the baby is a 'tight fit' for the birth canal, she disputes the idea that human pregnancy is cut short due to evolutionary necessity, observing that our gestation is not particularly shorter than other primates, and that some other primates also have a 'tight fit' at birth as well as highly dependent newborns. In a 2012 paper, she put forward a new theory, known as the 'EGG' or 'energetics of gestation and fetal growth' hypothesis, and this theory applies to all mammals, not just humans.[8] Dunsworth suggests that birth is triggered by the metabolic rate of the mother rising to 2.1 times the normal rate, the point at which her body would no longer be able to sustain the demands of the growing fetus. Dunsworth is careful to point out though that she does not feel her hypothesis is the definitive answer: 'The EGG hypothesis may turn out to be too good to be true. We have to keep searching, keep collecting evidence,' she says. Nevertheless, her work encourages us to think of the female body as fit for purpose; length of gestation is nothing to do with our pelvis, which is the size it needs to be. Indeed, evolution could have made it larger if necessary, but it has not had to. And Dunsworth is highly aware of the feminist nature of her work: 'If one were so inclined, one might even say that women's hips are *more* adapted than men's, given selection did not just build them as keystones of bipedalism but also as gateways for the ever-evolving species,' she told me. 'Nevertheless the obstetric dilemma is subsumed into the medical tradition and it is helping to overestimate risk and to underestimate women's bodies. Women are not "compromised" and our bodies do not pose dilemmas to be solved. We are just as adapted as men, and all the proof you need is that we birthed all of them.'

In spite of Dunsworth's work in this field, the obstetric dilemma is still widely used to justify the need for medical intervention in birth. On the popular website Healthline, for example, an article asks, 'How do Doctors Treat Birth Canal Issues?'[9] and gives this answer: 'A cesarean delivery is a common method to treat birth canal issues. According to the American Pregnancy Association, one-third of all cesarean deliveries are performed because of failure to progress in labor.' Scientists at the University of Vienna in 2016[10] suggested that the reason more and more women are having caesareans is because, well . . . because we are having more caesareans, passing on our faulty genes for too-narrow-pelvises and too-big-babies that in the past would have been eradicated by natural selection – in other words, the death of the faulty-gened mother or baby. Rather than dying, we are not only having the audacity to live through birth but we are having babies when we are fat and old, to boot, so the whole rising caesarean rate really is completely women's fault, whichever way you look at it.

These widespread attitudes with their entrenched sexism always start from the premise of female inadequacy, and in doing so fail to ask the right questions – first and foremost, why is there so much disparity? Or, to put it in the words of so many new mothers, 'How come she had a blissful home birth, and I had three days of agony in the hospital that ended in traumatic surgery?' If women are not properly built to give birth, how come some seem to manage it just fine? And looking wider, if we blame women's pathology for 'birth canal issues,' then we don't have to ask difficult questions about maternal mortality on a global basis, including the disparity between rich and poor, the very high and rising rates of maternal death in the USA, or the far higher mortality rates among black and ethnic minority women across the developed world. More black women die in childbirth, say some doctors, because they are at higher risk of complications such as pre-eclampsia, failing to address the institutionalised racism that also puts them at risk. Once again, women get the blame, and social injustice, as well as 'the system,' is off the hook.

# The evidence maze

When we are building our approach to birth on a bedrock of pathology rather than normality, of fear rather than confidence, there are a multitude of knock-on effects, many of which we all simply accept as 'how it goes,' just as we have all accepted the obstetric dilemma for over fifty years without question. Maternity care as we know it has developed in response to an underlying anxiety about the ability of women's bodies to work, and many interventions have been introduced on this basis, rather than on any firm scientific evidence. We now find ourselves in a place where we are required to produce evidence that accepted interventions *don't* work, in order to effect changes in practice. For example, the routine shave and enema had to be researched and found ineffective before it stopped happening to women, and currently, the practice of immediate cord clamping is slowly being phased out in the same way – although there was never a shred of evidence to support it in the first place.

'Evidence-based care' is a term many of us are familiar with, but. of course, not all evidence is created equal. In the UK, the Royal

College of Obstetricians and Gynaecologists (RCOG) addresses this by grading their guidelines according to how strong the evidence they are based on actually is.[11] Grade A is the label they give to what they consider to be top-quality evidence, usually based on a Randomised Controlled Trial (RCT).* Grades B and C are based on less strong evidence like reviews of the existing literature on a topic, and finally Grade D is given to the guidelines based on case reports and expert opinion. However, and this may shock you, only around 9 per cent of RCOG guidelines are based on Grade A evidence; 50 per cent of their guidelines are rated Grade B, C or D. Hang on a minute, I hear you say! Doesn't that leave 41 per cent without a grade at all? Yes, your maths is correct, and this is because they are not based on any evidence whatsoever, but rather on the opinions and experience of those who develop them. While their opinions and experience may indeed be sound, it's nevertheless important for pregnant women to know that they may wish to ask more questions about the grade or quality of the 'evidence base' for the recommendations they are receiving. And if so many recommendations are based on personal opinion and experience, do we also need to ask more questions about the fears, life experiences and assumptions of the people making these recommendations, which must surely be a powerful influence?

---

\* In an RCT people are randomly allocated to two or more groups, with one group having the intervention, and the other not. As you can imagine, RCTs are difficult to undertake in maternity care as many women do not wish for their birth choices to be 'randomised' in this way.

We also need to consider that the more medicalised childbirth becomes, the more we may lose track of any sense of 'normality' when we are researching the best way to go about it. The widely reported 2018 ARRIVE[12] trial is a case in point. The trial found that routine induction at 39 weeks *reduced* the chance of caesarean (from 22 per cent to 18 per cent), which was hailed by many as a breakthrough which could pave the way to routine inductions at 39 weeks for all women as standard.[13] But this research took place in America and simply compared highly medicalised induced births with highly medicalised non-induced births – only 6 per cent of participants were cared for by a midwife, for example.[14] As birth expert Henci Goer puts it, 'The trial is nothing more than a frying pan vs. fire comparison with the not surprising finding that in the hands of medical-model practitioners, the frying pan comes out slightly ahead of the fire.'[15] The possibility of a 'third way' – in which women's natural physiology is respected and they receive one to one support from a midwife they trust – was not part of the trial's comparison. And as this way of birth becomes more and more rare, it will surely feature in less and less research, leaving only the frying pan and the fire to be compared and studied.

## Have you had that baby yet?

Induction itself is a hot topic. In modern maternity care systems, around 25 per cent of women now have their labour 'induced'.[16] And this keeps steeply rising – 2018 figures in England show that 32 per cent of women are induced, that's 1 in 3 labours being started artificially, compared to 1 in 5 just ten years previously.[17] In some settings in the UK, USA and Australia, that rate can be even higher, as much as 45 per cent The most common reason for induction is being 'post dates,' and as pregnant women across the globe will tell you, the anxiety around going past your due date usually begins long before you even get near it. Discussions about induction can start at around 37 or 38 weeks, and at this point there will often be offers of a friendly 'membrane sweep' from your midwife, 'just to see if we can get things moving!' – for this read, 'if they don't get moving, you'll end up being induced'. There is some evidence that sweeps may start your labour and thus make medical induction less likely, but a Cochrane review highlights adverse effects such as discomfort, bleeding and irregular contractions, and estimates that 8 women will have to be 'swept' to avoid one induction.[18] Avoidance of induction, though, is often what those last weeks of pregnancy are all about, and alongside sweeps, there are literally hundreds of thousands of internet articles devoted to 'natural induction methods,' with pregnant women frantically eating pineapples, running upstairs sideways and even drinking castor oil in an effort to go into labour 'on time'.

At this point I should probably declare that I was one of those women. When I had my first baby in 2008, I tried literally everything I could to get my body to go into labour, although none of it worked and I was induced at 42 weeks and 3 days. My next two babies were born at home, with no attempts to bring on labour whatsoever, both at 42 weeks on the dot – it seems like I am just a 'slow cooker' and 42 weeks is 'normal' for me. In fact, I think my first baby would have turned up sooner if I *hadn't* been so anxious and desperate for labour to start – and I had had the confidence of my care providers, too. Instead, it felt like everyone around me doubted my ability to do even the most basic 'entry level' task of childbirth – and this really fed my fears that I was not going to be up to the main job at all. I was given a membrane sweep *four times*. These were painful, undignified and unpleasant, especially the last one. Having drunk castor oil that day to explosive effect, I'd spent the afternoon crapping through the eye of yet another pesky proverbial needle, and turned up at the hospital to be monitored in the midst of some quite nice, regular contractions, a good sign of early labour. I was 42 weeks, on the dot. Before I left, the midwife said, 'I'm just going to give you one last sweep, and I'm really going to *go for it* this time.' It was horrific, my partner heard my yelps from outside the room, and added to this, my contractions stopped and that was the last I saw of them until I was induced a few days later. My personal view is that my cervix slammed shut like a clam shell and would have been better left alone at this point – but I can't prove this scientifically of course – it's just how I feel about what happened to my body that day. The midwife who did the sweep had good intentions – as I left the hospital she said cheerfully, 'Go home and have your baby!' Everyone knew I wanted a home birth and that it was against policy to have one if I went past 42 weeks. Grandfather Time was master of all of us that day, it seemed, as it is of so many women who feel that, even before they reach their due date, the clock is ticking, and they must beat it.

Because the due date itself is tied up in most people's consciousness with the ultramodern ultrasound scan, many people perceive the prediction of when the baby will show up to be high tech and therefore accurate and reliable. In reality, the whole system is based on a seventeenth-century calculation method which to this day, nobody is really quite sure about. If we are going to talk about 'evidence-based' maternity care we could do worse than start with asking why the modern world still calculates pregnancy length using 'Naegele's rule,' named after the German professor who suggested that you work the whole thing out by adding seven days to the last menstrual period, and then adding nine months. As well as the fact that this theory in itself was based on research by someone called Boerhaave that involved the records of just 100 pregnant women – not exactly large-scale research – the other problem with Naegele's rule is that nobody has ever been clear if he meant that you should add seven days to the first day or the last day of the last period. In the 1900s, American textbooks ran with adding it to the first day of the last period, and this is where we have stayed ever since, with almost all doctors, midwives and health professionals calculating due dates using this somewhat shaky maths.[19]

Prior to scientific attempts to calculate due dates, women are thought to have expected to give birth within ten moon cycles of their last period – around 295 days, or 42 weeks. Naegele's formula shortens this to 280 days, or 40 weeks.[20] This two-week difference may seem relatively small but when you are waiting for a baby, it is key to both your own expectations and those of your care providers, affecting the way that both you and they behave and feel. And while it's wrong to suggest that due dates are complete rubbish, it might be fair to say that we need to have more of a degree of flexibility around them than we do currently. Ultrasound due dates may be slightly more accurate than those calculated on the dates of your last period but, ultimately, the chance of a baby being born on their due date is less than 5 per cent.[21] Perhaps we'd all be a lot better following the royal example and having a 'due month,' since the majority of babies will turn up any time between 38 and 42 weeks. There is evidence that induction after 41 weeks reduces the chance of stillbirth,[22] but leading bodies like Cochrane and NICE offer very measured advice on this: 'Women with uncomplicated pregnancies should be given every opportunity to go into spontaneous labour [and] should usually be offered induction of labour between 41+0 and 42+0 weeks to avoid the risks of prolonged pregnancy. The exact timing should take into account the woman's preferences and local circumstances. If a woman chooses not to have induction of labour, her decision should be respected' say NICE,[23] and Cochrane says, 'Births after 42 weeks' gestation may slightly increase risks for babies, including a greater risk of death (before or shortly after birth). However, induction of labour may also have risks for mothers and their babies, especially if women are not ready to labour. No tests can predict if babies would be better to stay inside their mother or if labour should be induced to make the birth happen sooner.' These laid-back attitudes don't seem to translate to women's actual experiences, though, with many reporting that they don't feel they are presented with a real choice, and that the pressure starts mounting from about week 37.

Women frequently report to me that the use of 'assertions' can begin long before their due date, for example, 'If you don't go into labour by x weeks, we will induce you.' Some say they are given 'soundbites' such as being told, 'Your risk of stillbirth doubles after 42 weeks,' without any further information about what this really means, what evidence it is based on, or what the actual risk may be for them personally. Women rarely report any discussion or acknowledgement of the risks of induction but feel that the emphasis is always on the risk of continuing to be pregnant. Many feel under pressure, 'like a ticking time bomb,' with several reporting being told that their placenta would soon fail, or even that it is probably already failing. Others describe how they feel they literally cannot decline the induction appointment, but are instead urged to 'make the appointment and then don't turn up if you are still against it'. Some report being given a cursory leaflet; many say they were told 'It's policy to induce you' without being offered information about any alternative paths. I could fill another book with such stories. Emma, who gave birth in Sussex in 2018, told me, 'I was automatically booked in for an induction despite my refusal, because "we always induce at 40 + 8". No one explained anything to me about it at all, it was just assumed that I would go along with it, and I met a lot of negativity and cajoling when I kept refusing. But still no one explained anything, they just said "so you want to put your baby at risk then". It was not a nice experience.' Caitlin from Leicestershire, who gave birth in 2016, reported similar: 'I knew the precise date of my conception but was told that I was wrong and the scan was right. At my 40-week appointment the midwife just picked up the phone and booked me in at the hospital.' And Laura, who holds a BSc in Biology from Durham, was asked by her consultant, 'What do you think the "so-called" risks of induction are then?' When she told him, he replied, 'And where did you get that from? Netmums?'

I think it's important that we see this as two separate debates that sometimes get conflated: yes, we need to continue to understand more about the evidence for induction, the causes of stillbirth and how we may prevent it, and yes, we also need to consider the ways that we are currently presenting maternity risks and choices to women. Even if the benefits of induction at 41 weeks or even earlier are found to be extremely strong, women should still be given balanced information based on their personal situation, be listened to and spoken to with respect, and ultimately be able to decline as well as accept what is often a highly medicalised experience.

More research is needed, and this should focus on long-term effects of induction as well as possible impacts on women's choices, the 'cons' as well as the 'pros'. Too often women are given false impressions or blanket statements about the certainty of our current understanding, which can leave them feeling anxious about the safety of their baby in utero or even feeling that their womb itself is a hostile place that it would be better for their baby to leave. Question marks also hang over the reputation of the placenta, which will often be talked about in terms of its 'deterioration' and its 'ageing,' while in fact there is no clear evidence to support the idea that placentas 'age,' or to link any cellular changes in the placenta with stillbirth past 42 weeks. There is evidence that the structure and biochemistry of the placenta changes as it ages but while this is viewed by some as evidence of deterioration, others see it in more positive terms – as adaptation to the changing baby. Some suggest this speculation over its shelf-life is yet another myth about the poor design of the female body. Writing in 1997,[24] renowned histopathologist and placenta expert Professor Harold Fox said that there was 'no logical reason to believe that the placenta, which is a fetal organ, should age while the other fetal organs do not,' adding that you don't find a situation where an individual organ ages, within an organism that is not aged, in any other biological system. The whole concept of 'placental insufficiency,' said Fox, was facile and had been too readily accepted. Hmm. That sounds familiar.

Rising rates of induction mean rising rates of medicalised birth – in spite of the repeated claims that induction makes birth safer, it's unusual to have a home birth or a birth centre birth if you are induced, due to being 'higher risk'. While being 'post dates' is the biggest reason for starting labour artificially, women are also induced for suspected big babies, for 'advanced maternal age' (most often interpreted as being past 40 weeks and over 40 years old), for gestational diabetes, for waters breaking with no other signs of labour, and for other health concerns about the welfare of mother or baby. The explanation for the recent sudden up-tick in induction rates across the developed world is usually wide-sweeping: 'mothers are getting older and fatter,'[25] and while it's true that giving birth later in life or having a higher BMI can increase the chance of complications, induction rates seem to be rising across the population – young, slim women are induced too. In the UK, for example, where almost 30 per cent of women are induced, RCOG recommends induction for anyone over 40, which makes up just 4 per cent of pregnant women. Induction is just one of the many examples of a pregnancy minefield – while some health concerns may be well founded, if you are a pregnant woman in the trenches of antenatal decision making, it can be very hard to discern which apply to you, what the actual risks are, and what the evidence base is for the advice you are being given. In the case of induction, for example, you may be told that labour will be more painful or more likely to end in intervention, while others may say this is not the case at all. You will also find plenty of anecdotal evidence of both positive and negative experiences of induction, making it even harder to decide what to do. This is not to say that all research is worthless, but rather that there is a lot of it out there, and it can be hard to find studies that actually apply to your specific circumstances or to know which research is the best quality. If a particular course of action is being recommended to you, you may like to ask your midwife or doctor, 'On what specific evidence is this recommendation based?' (ask for a link). If they are happy to discuss the research with you, ask, 'When did this research take place? What kind of research was it? How does this research apply to me in my specific situation? And is there any other evidence that might be relevant to me as I make my choice?' (again, get a link).

# FINDING THE EVIDENCE

When faced with a decision in maternity care, try the BRAIN acronym. Ask:

B – What are the benefits?

R – What are the risks?

A – What are the alternatives?

I – What is my intuition telling me?

N – What happens if we do nothing?

You can also do your own research to find out what the existing evidence has to say about your choices. Here are some starting points for good resources.

**Your health care provider.** The person recommending a certain course of action should be able to point you to the evidence upon which this suggestion is based.

**NICE guidelines.** These guidelines are put together by teams of academics, professionals and service users, are based on the best available evidence, and are regularly reviewed and revised. NICE is a UK public body and part of the Department of Health; however, practitioners in many other parts of the world look to NICE to find the best standards of practice, so, if you are reading this book and are beyond the UK, you may still find NICE guidelines useful and highly applicable to your situation. Particularly useful is CG190. Search 'NICE CG190' or 'NICE guideline ____' and fill in the blank with the issue you need

more information about. Alternatively visit www.rcog.org.uk/
guidelines and use their search box – select NICE guidelines in
the drop-down menu.

> *Giving birth is a life-changing event. The care that
> a woman receives during labour has the potential to
> affect her – both physically and emotionally, in the
> short and longer term – and the health of her baby.
> Good communication, support and compassion from
> staff, and having her wishes respected, can help her
> feel in control of what is happening and contribute to
> making birth a positive experience for the woman and
> her birth companion(s).*

> Extract from the Introduction to NICE Clinical
> Guideline 190

**Cochrane reviews.** Cochrane reviews are internationally
recognised as the highest standard in evidence-based health
care resources. Search for 'Cochrane review _____' and fill
in the blank with the issue you want to know more about, e.g.
'Cochrane review induction of labour'. Alternatively visit www.
cochranelibrary.com and use the search box.

**RCOG Green-top guidelines.** Guidelines for UK obstetricians on
pretty much every pregnancy and birth scenario.

Visit www.rcog.org.uk/guidelines and use their brilliant search
facility, either to search the Green-top Guidelines, or explore the
drop-down menu to find other guidelines and reports, including
the NICE guidelines.

**ACOG and SOGC.** The American College of Obstetricians and Gynecologists (ACOG) and the Society of Obstetricians and Gynecologists of Canada (SOGC) have practice bulletins and guidelines that can be found at www.acog.org/Resources-And-Publications/Practice-Bulletins-List
and www.jogc.com/clinical-practice-guidelines
respectively.

**Which? Birth Choice.** Want to know how your local hospital compares to the national average when it comes to everything from numbers of caesareans to your chances of having stitches? Find information about where to give birth and a wide range of stats on all of your nearest units, searchable by postcode at www.which.co.uk/birth-choice.

**Bump2Babe.** Consumer guide to Irish maternity care with clear stats on every hospital and lots of information about your choices. www.bump2babe.ie/

**Evidence Based Birth.** American website written by researcher Rebecca Dekker, which gives a really accessible overview of the evidence relating to many of the major birth choices and dilemmas. www.evidencebasedbirth.com

Researchers are also out of the habit of finding out something pretty vital: how do women 'feel' about this? What was their experience? Many induction studies, for example, take us back into the 'frying pan' vs. 'fire' zone, simply comparing the outcomes of 'induced' with 'not induced' and failing to ask questions about the type of care women received, or how they felt about their birth experience beyond the rather dry concept of 'satisfaction'. Just as the Victorian woman who lay on her back during sex and hoped it would soon be over probably had no idea what she was missing, so too a generation or two of birthing women have very little to compare things to, when and if they are asked to rate how they felt about it. Ultimately, though, women's birth experience is not thought to be important in comparison to the very admirable current drive to reduce stillbirth and other poor outcomes in labour and birth, and because women's decisions are usually framed around the risk of these tragic occurrences, everyone in the conversation – even the woman herself – collectively and willingly shunts feelings into the background. Nobody could argue that tealights and a reiki massage trump everyone getting out alive – it's a no-brainer.

Safety is the justification for induction as it is for most other birth interventions, but there often appears to be much less discussion of any relationship between adverse outcomes and induction itself – it is consistently presented as a way to *avoid* harm to mother or baby and there is rarely discussion of whether it could *cause* harm – either in the short or long term. Does it increase the risk of pelvic floor damage? What about birth trauma, is this higher in induced women? What about breastfeeding rates? And newborn bonding? What about women's self-esteem, or body image, following induction? And how about the baby's long-term health? There seems to be very little data and certainly most or all of these questions are not discussed with pregnant women to whom induction is being recommended. One study has found that synthetic oxytocin in labour (which is not exclusive to induction – some women have it to speed up their labour even if it has started spontaneously) may increase the risk of postnatal depression by as much as 32 per cent.[26] Another study has found higher rates of respiratory infections, metabolic disorders and eczema among children whose births included medical intervention, including induction.[27] In Australia, Professor John Newnham, a leading expert in maternal and fetal medicine who runs a campaign called The Whole Nine Months to prevent preterm birth, has spoken out about the practice of early induction, either to prevent stillbirth or simply for the convenience of parents or doctors' schedules, and highlighted the need for balance.[28] He points to the long-term consequences for neurodevelopment in babies born prior to 39 weeks, and puts it starkly: 'If you had a hypothetical school of 500 children and with each class having 30 children, if you electively delivered all the children at 37 weeks rather than later, you may have one extra child in the school (by preventing one stillbirth) but you would expect to have two extra children in each class of 30 with externalising behavioural problems, and every second class would have an extra child with requirements for special educational assistance.' While he acknowledges the importance of stillbirth prevention, he points out that other risks can be left out of the early induction conversation. 'If mothers went back to their obstetrician and said, "See this kid behaving poorly at school, this is your fault", it would stop immediately. But that doesn't happen,' he says, 'The obstetrician is only focused on death, and they are not focused on the school-aged children.'[29]

## Measuring up

If we would only accept that women's bodies are not very good at giving birth, then we would very quickly see that it is women, and their high expectations, that are in dire need of adjustment – well, seemingly according to a study in May 2018 from Irish researchers who chose the witty title, 'How would Mary Poppins fare in labour? Practically perfect? Unlikely.'[30] I'm guessing that they were referring to the Julie Andrews version of this famous character, notoriously despised by Poppins's outspoken and fiercely feminist creator, Pamela Lyndon Travers, who felt that the Disney film presented a dumbed-down, saccharine version of her original, much darker and multi-dimensional heroine. Defining a 'practically perfect' birth as a labour without intervention, and with an intact perineum and a positive neonatal outcome, the researchers concluded that out of the 8,292 Irish first-time mothers they studied, only 0.8 per cent had this Poppins-style experience. They felt their findings had great implications for how we talk to pregnant women about what to expect, since, to use their exact words, 'Unrealistic expectations of labour in first-time mothers can present challenges to physicians and midwives.' The subtext of this suggests that women with low expectations of birth are much less 'demanding' and therefore easier for professionals to engage with and manage. Perhaps they even gave away their unconscious desires in the title of their study, casting themselves as Julie Andrews and strictly measuring the women in their care, accepting no nonsense, and bringing order and conformity with a click of their fingers. Be a bit more Disney and a bit less P.L. Travers, girls, because Nanny knows best.

As Poppins herself would tell you, though, the results you get depend precisely upon what you measure. Of course, if you look at a large group of predominantly hospital birthers, you will find that they had very medicalised experiences. You could extrapolate from that that women's bodies don't work very well and that we should all adjust our expectations of birth accordingly. On the other hand, you could try measuring something different. The world was somewhat shocked in 2011, when the National Perinatal Epidemiology Unit at the University of Oxford published the results of a wide-scale study examining the impact of the planned place of birth for women who were 'low risk'. The Birthplace study[31] looked at over 60,000 women and told us that, first and foremost, giving birth in the UK is very safe. However, the part that some people still struggle to accept nearly a decade later is that they also found that, for low-risk women, it was *safer* to plan to give birth at home or in a midwife-led unit (MLU) than it was to plan to birth in an obstetric unit, in terms of avoiding major medical interventions. Caesareans, instrumental births, episiotomies, third- or fourth-degree tears, the need for blood transfusion and the need for admission to intensive care, happened much less frequently to women who planned a birth at home or in a birth centre. For those having their first baby, Birthplace found that home birth, while still better for the mother, was slightly less safe for the baby, with the chance of an adverse outcome (stillbirth or serious harm) rising from 5 in 1,000 in an obstetric unit to 9 in 1,000 for planned home births. For second-time mums and beyond, home birth was just as safe for the baby. Looking at the Birthplace stats[32] you can clearly see that to get closer to a 'practically perfect' birth, rather than lower your expectations, you might be better off choosing a different door – or simply staying put behind your own. Birth is not pot luck, and women's bodies 'work better' according to the choices they make. This message was not so easy for the world to swallow, however, and Peter Brocklehurst, then Professor of Perinatal Epidemiology at Oxford and the Birthplace principal investigator, described it as, 'the most controversial piece of research I've ever done'.[33] The press spin on the study was also interesting, often focusing exclusively on outcomes for babies and ignoring women, emphasising only negative findings, and exaggerating the extent of the difference for babies. Many papers chose to lead with the potential negative impact for the baby of home birth for a first-time mother, with headlines like, 'Home birth three times more risky than hospital, says study' (*Metro*, 24 November 2011)[34] and 'First-time mothers who opt for home birth face triple the risk of death or brain damage in child' (*Daily Mail*, 25 November 2011).[35] This total twist on the facts of the Birthplace study reinforced to women that they were better off in hospital even when a highly regarded piece of research had just found otherwise. This is the patriarchal machine in full motion, cutting women off from information that might be empowering to them, reminiscent of the Peel Report,[36] a parliamentary review in 1970, that called for 100 per cent hospital delivery, and is credited with the dramatic increase in this option, with 91.4 per cent of women birthing in hospital by 1972, up from 68.2 in 1963. 'The greater safety of hospital confinement for mother and child justifies this objective,' said the report, which based this claim on absolutely zero evidence and asked not a single woman for her views or preferences.

We can also look at stats from care providers who 'do things differently' – and this often means that a faith and confidence in women's bodies to 'work' underpins their practice. Bronwyn Moir was a hospital midwife in New South Wales, Australia, before setting up her own private practice and a home-from-home setting for women who live a long distance from the hospital, called the Lismore Birth House.[37] 'I have a lot more faith in the ability of women's bodies since working as a home birth midwife,' she told me. 'I had to do a lot of unlearning and unpacking of my own conditioned fears, coming out of working within the hospital setting.' Over the past five years Bronwyn has cared for 115 pregnant women, and 89 per cent of them have gone on to have normal, vaginal births, the majority of them at home or in the birth house. Only 6 per cent of the women she has cared for have gone on to have a caesarean, and only 5 per cent have had instrumental deliveries. The women in her care are both 'high risk' and 'low risk' – including three sets of twins, women with gestational diabetes, high BMI, over the age of 45, VBAC and other potential complications.

What is she doing differently? Quite a lot, it seems – although a lot of the difference rests with what she is *not* doing. None of the women in her care have ever been induced, although she does recommend extra monitoring if people go post-dates, and discussion of the risks and choices with an obstetrician if they get to 42 weeks. She does not do routine vaginal exams in labour or use time as a factor in decision making. 'In both the first and second stage, as long as there is some form of progress and the woman and the baby are stable, we keep going. It's usually the woman who calls it during a really long labour when she wants pain relief and we transfer to hospital. Of the 18 per cent of women who transfer to hospital, 48 per cent will still go on to have a normal vaginal birth.'

Bronwyn thinks the explanation for her amazing results is simple. 'The most obvious reason for the good stats is the continuity of carer and relationship-based care. A typical birth at the Lismore Birth House, or at home, is usually private, dark and undisturbed. We talk a lot during pregnancy about the effect the environment can have on birthing hormones and we do birth planning to allow space for women to really think about who they want in their birth space. We try to do lots of education with partners and support team so that everyone knows how best to support physiological birth. As midwives at a birth, we try to support the woman through comfort measures but ultimately we just try to not disturb her.'

## Hands off!

Undisturbed birth, that ability to keep in the background and 'sit on your hands,' seems to be key. Some midwives refer to this as 'intelligent tea drinking,' or 'intuitive crochet'. Being present, relaxed, trusting in the process of birth, holding the space for the woman but keeping a distance until needed, is considered by some to be the art of midwifery. I asked midwife Becky Reed to give her persepective on this: 'I think the skill lies in knowing when to do nothing (which is most of the time!) and when to do something,' she told me. 'And of course, if the midwife knows the woman that makes everything so much easier. Most births will go smoothly if the woman feels safe, and if her baby is in a good position and labour has started by itself. In those births the midwife needs to do very little – stay in tune with the labouring woman and make sure any actions (e.g. talking, listening to the baby's heartbeat) are appropriate and feel right for the mother. And give off an aura of positivity.' She went on to say that 'Sometimes the baby is in a difficult position and labour doesn't progress easily, and then it might be appropriate to intervene (with the mother's agreement and working together) to help things along. And that's the intelligent bit – keeping quietly watchful and knowing when to act or not to act.' This kind of 'hands-off' maternity care is currently fading into the history books, but might we be missing some very tangible benefits? At the moment, the RCOG are rightly concerned about the rising rates of perineal damage at birth. Serious tears during childbirth can cause problems long after a baby is born, even for a lifetime, including incontinence – both urinary and fecal – and sexual dysfunction. According to the RCOG, most women – around 90 per cent – will tear during childbirth[38] – it seems like the perineum is yet another part of the female body that 'can't be relied on to do its job properly' – but only a very small percentage will sustain the severe damage known as third- and fourth-degree tears, or Severe Perineal Tears (SPT). Between 2000 and 2012, the rate of SPTs in England has tripled from 1.8 per cent to 5.9 per cent among first-time mothers.[39]

Let's compare that stat to those of the Albany where Becky Reed practised, first of all. From 1997 to 2009 they provided care to over 2,500 women, and their rates of perineal damage were minimal. Two-thirds of women (62.2 per cent) who had a vaginal birth had no damage at all, 13.3 per cent a first-degree tear, and 19.8 per cent a second-degree tear. Just sixteen of the women they attended had a third-degree tear – 0.7 per cent – and there were no fourth-degree tears.[40] So, let's just recap that: the RCOG says that 90 per cent of women will sustain some perineal damage during childbirth, but at the Albany, fewer than 40 per cent did. And the current rate of SPT in England is roughly eight times higher than the Albany – who also had no fourth-degree tears at all.

How about the Lismore Birth House? Well, 51 per cent of women who birthed under their care had a completely intact perineum, 19 per cent had first-degree tears and 25 per cent had second-degree tears. Similar to the Albany, only 0.85 per cent had a third-degree tear (which represents 1 out of 117 births), and their only fourth-degree tear occurred at a forceps delivery with episiotomy after a hospital transfer. What do they do at the Lismore? 'We talk a lot about it during pregnancy, what can help give them the best chance of not tearing, for example, good nutrition, position at birth, perineal massage during pregnancy, and slow birth of the head,' Bronwyn Moir told me. 'I'm completely hands off at the birth,

I just give verbal guidance to slow down the crowning part. I may suggest that a woman puts her own hands on her baby's head to get a feel of how fast they are coming and help her to instinctively slow it down. I offer warm compresses on the perineum, though a lot of women are in the pool, so that does the same thing. I don't do any coached pushing.'

The stats of world-famous midwife Ina May Gaskin, whose 'Farm' midwifery centre bears similarities in set-up and ethos to the Lismore, are the best of the lot. 'Obstetricians of earlier generations planted the idea (that is still widely held) that nature cheated women . . . and that their crotches are made of shoddy goods,' twinkles Ina in her *Guide to Childbirth*. She argues for engorgement in childbirth, the same kind that we experience during sexual arousal, and believes that the majority of women are 'well equipped to give birth without the slightest injury'. Her figures bear this out, over 40 years, 68.7 per cent of women in her care gave birth with an intact perineum, 19.4 per cent had a first-degree tear, 3.2 per cent had a second-degree tear, 0.3 per cent had a third-degree tear and 0.04 per cent had a fourth-degree tear.[41]

> *Men take it for granted that their sexual organs can greatly increase in size and then become small again without being ruined. If obstetricians (and women) could understand that women's genitals have similar abilities, episiotomy and laceration rates might go down overnight.*
>
> Ina May Gaskin, *Ina May's Guide to Childbirth*[42]

# Hands on

For those women who do experience severe tears in childbirth, this can be the beginning of a lifetime of continence issues or a sex life that is never the same again. Women who experience this damage often feel that their concerns are not properly addressed in the postnatal period, and there are valid calls for much better advice, checks and physiotherapy for women who have just given birth. The RCOG and RCM in the UK, and the Women's Health Authority (WHA) in Australia, responded in 2018 by trialling very similar 'care bundles' to try to reduce the current rising rates of tearing. Nobody knows the reason for the rise, although there is speculation that, yes, you've guessed it, it's because birthing women are older and fatter. The 'care bundle,' known as the 'OASI care bundle'\* in the UK, is being trialled in 16 maternity units, and involves several elements, which ideally should all be implemented together for optimal effect. These are: 'speaking with the woman about her risk and OASI and communicating with her during the birth to enable a slow controlled birth of the baby, performing an episiotomy (a cut in the perineum to assist birth and prevent tears) when required, using the hands to enable perineal protection at

---

\*    RCOG and other professional bodies refers to third- and fourth-degree tears as OASI or OASIS (obstetric anal sphincter injuries), but some women who have experienced these injuries object to the acronym and the associated image of an oasis, which bears no relation to their suffering. For this reason, in this book third- and fourth-degree tears are referred to as SPT or severe perineal trauma wherever possible.

the time of birth and a thorough examination after birth to detect tears'.[43]

The final two points on the list are of key interest. Firstly, the 'hands on' perineal protection is something quite specific called the Finnish Grip. If you are interested to know more about this you can search 'Finnish Grip OASI' in YouTube and you will find the demonstration video[44] – a disembodied lower torso with an emerging baby, in the lithotomy position, with one gloved hand making a 'V' with their fingers at the base of the vagina, while the other hand pushes on the baby's emerging head to slow delivery, which is entirely verbally guided by the person doing the grip. As someone who has seen and heard so many examples of hands-off, upright birth – and experienced two such births personally – I must admit I watched with horror.

The second point of interest is the post-birth examination, which, if you are a professional who is participating in the care bundle, you are expected to do after every single vaginal delivery, even if there is a completely intact perineum. This examination involves a finger inserted into the anus to check above the sphincter, and then withdrawn slowly while placing the thumb in the vagina as the anal sphincter is palpated 'from 9 to 3 o'clock'.[45] If you suspect damage you may call a second clinician who will perform the same check. A woman's consent must of course be sought for this, but how much explicit detail she is given about which fingers are going to go where and do what is unclear. Nor is it clear how this consent can be completely 'informed consent,' since, while women with tearing will always have had this exam to assess the severity – and probably welcomed it because when something is wrong you do actually need a doctor – it's a new proposition entirely for all women to have it even if their perineum is intact. There don't seem to be any available statistics on the incidence of women who have 'hidden' tears in spite of looking perfectly OK from the outside.[46] Nor is there any clarity on what the advantage may be to early detection of these hidden injuries. Nor is there information on the number of women who would need to have the exam in order to prevent one missed diagnosis. Obstetrics professor Jim Thornton has said, 'The idea of such an intrusive procedure, at such a sensitive time, makes no sense. Routine rectal examination in the presence of an intact perineum fails all the criteria of a useful screening test.'[47] And yet without full information about the benefits and risks of an exam, and without also being told what the possible consequence of a missed diagnosis may be, how can a woman with an intact perineum weigh up whether or not she wants the exam? Is this informed consent?

Of course, there are other, clearer consequences of a missed tear: litigation. On their introductory information for doctors and midwives about the bundle, the Royal College of Obstetricians is straightforward about this: 'Damage to the anal sphincter must be ruled out for every woman who has a vaginal birth. Failure to do this is the leading cause of negligence claims amongst women who present with "missed" third- or fourth-degree tears. Compensation for women varies according to their symptoms, but recent cases show that it is approximately £200,000.'[48] There is an element of 'self-protection' in 'perineal protection' it seems.

None of this is to diminish the awful consequences of perineal damage, especially if it goes undetected. But we do need to ask questions about why the current attempt at addressing this problem seems, yet again, to devalue the woman's personal experience in the quest for safety. There has been no discussion, for example, of research that has found women who plan home births – a way of birthing that many women also really enjoy – to have lower incidents of perineal trauma.[49] The Finnish Grip – as demonstrated in the video – is easiest for the clinician if the woman is on her back, and impossible if she is upright or in water. It's of dubious value if she is on all fours, as one midwife put it to me, 'We are told to "Do it the same but upside down", so how does me leaving my hand on the perineum above the fetal head prevent the shoulder pressure on the perineum? It doesn't.' Midwives keen to comply with the 'OASI bundle' may well be tempted to encourage women out of pools or onto their backs, for optimum effect. Nor is it clear whether a 'hands on' approach during childbirth prevents tearing at all – a 2017 Cochrane review (considered by most to be the best evidence) found the evidence inconclusive either way and recommended more research.[50] Anecdotally, the Finnish Grip may even be *causing* tears – I've heard from several midwives who are concerned it simply redirects pressure to the clitoral area and is causing damage there instead. If we were to be really cynical, we might also speculate that clitoral tears will cause less litigation than anal ones, since a woman's sexual experience is less tangible and also less culturally valued than her continence.

As it stands, then, women are getting a highly interventionist birth experience in which they are likely to be birthing on beds, on their backs, rarely upright or in a birth pool, often under epidural and under time pressure, unsupported by someone they know, told when and how to push and rarely encouraged to listen to their body and instinct. After this, a routine exam of their two most intimate orifices comes in an attempt to fix a problem that is potentially caused by the very system trying to solve it. There is absolutely zero introspection here. Instead, in a mostly unspoken way, it's implied that women and their bodies are the cause of the problem, rather than anything that is being done *to* them. And the solution? Do more *to* them. No mention is made of birth positions, physiology, environment, continuity of carer, water birth, place of birth, perineal massage or any other possible way of preventing tears that might be woman-centred or involve the carers *not* doing something, rather than doing something. As midwifery academic Dr Rachel Reed put it to me, 'These interventions have been introduced in an attempt to deal with all the damage other interventions are doing to women's perineums. If care providers supported physiology they wouldn't have to "protect" women's perineums. It is just another reflection of mistrust of women and their bodies.'

## Technologised mistrust

There are so many other areas of what I am going to call 'technologised mistrust'. Here are a few to consider, and once you turn your attention to these, you may find yourself noticing many more.

**Why does Continuous Electronic Fetal Monitoring (CEFM) continue to be used in spite of zero evidence to support it?** Being strapped to a machine to monitor your contractions and your baby's heartbeat (also known as a CTG) will happen to you if there are concerns about you or your baby, before or during labour, and in the USA and some other countries, you will get CEFM as standard. However, there is no evidence that it improves outcomes apart from possibly reducing the very rare chance of neonatal seizures. On the other hand, it is associated with a significantly higher rate of caesarean and instrumental delivery,[51] perhaps in part due to its false positive rate of around 60 per cent,[52] meaning that it often highlights non-existent problems. CTGs that are given without any indication to all women on admission to hospital (as happens in the USA, for example) have been shown to increase the caesarean rate by about 20 per cent.[53] If you are offered CEFM but you don't want to be on a bed on your back, you can ask for 'wireless telemetry' or even a waterproof version for a pool birth, but you may be lucky to get it, since these machines, and people who know how to operate them, are apparently as rare as hen's teeth.

**Speaking of water birth, why are there safety concerns about it?** Well that's a very good question. The ACOG (American College of Obstetricians and Gynecologists) is really opposed to water birth, stating possible dangers, insisting that women should get out for the birth itself, and adding that there is not enough evidence that water birth has any 'maternal benefit'.[54] I'm not sure which water-birthing women they spoke to in order to arrive at that conclusion, but I've only ever heard women describe the benefits in evangelical terms.

In the UK there's a softer attitude to birth in the pool but it's still harder than you think to get access to one in labour, and even harder actually to give birth in one, especially if you are 'high risk' – only around 1 in 10 UK women deliver their babies in water.[55] There are still regular spates[56] of alarmist headlines[57] about how it might be risky, although there don't seem to be similar levels of media concern about CEFM, or indeed, about the 'OASI care bundle'.

> *Water birth like home birth is controversial. Why?*
> *Because the obstetricians are out of control. It's that*
> *simple. The water helps the woman, but it sure doesn't*
> *help the birth attendant. It's the opposite of the*
> *lithotomy position, which helps the birth attendant, but*
> *doesn't help the woman.*
>
> Marsden Wagner[58]

**Why do we continue to watch the clock?** If we're not looking at the machinery surrounding the woman, we seem constantly to be checking the time, mainly worrying that she is 'taking too long' either to dilate or to push her baby out. You can feel this pressure yourself even in the throes of labour. The standard guideline is that we should all dilate neatly at 1cm per hour, but birth doesn't often conform to these norms, causing many health care professionals and even women themselves to worry that the female body is not working as it should, when in fact it's just doing what humans do – being unique.[59] The World Health Organisation has said that 'labour progress at 1cm per hour may be unrealistic for some' and that 'every birth is unique,' adding that, 'unnecessary medical interventions should be avoided if the mother and her baby are in good condition,' and this is based on evidence – as you would expect from the WHO.[60] Evidence about the length of the second stage is more complicated[61] – it's hard to get away from the land of frying pan and fire here, and work out how long women who have not had epidurals, are not placed on their backs, and are in supportive, woman-centred care, for example, might need to push their baby out – but it's still clear that setting an arbitrary time deadline is not personalised enough. And on that note …

**Why are we shouting at women to PUSH?** This is perhaps another symptom of the 'clock panic,' and also related to epidural use – you do actually need some help to know when and how to 'bear down' if you cannot feel any sensation below your waist. But this approach to giving birth has become so ingrained that it's literally the sit-com/soap 'go to' for the birth moment. You see it on reality shows too – on *One Born Every Minute* I once saw a midwife urge a woman to 'Get angry with your baby!' Perhaps she would be angry, if she knew about the fetal ejection reflex (FER) – a well-kept secret and a rather clunky term for a process that takes over a woman's body – but usually only in undisturbed, 'hands off' births.[62] FER means you don't actually have to 'push' at all – it all happens by itself – summed up to me brilliantly (and rather graphically!) by one woman who experienced it as 'reverse vomiting'. Some may welcome professional guidance for the moments of birth, others would prefer silence so they can focus – but women don't always get a choice. Nor are they always listened to …

**Why don't we believe women when they say they are in labour?** Or even, when they say they are about to have a baby? Women frequently report being turned away from the labour ward because they are 'not in labour' and this having a range of consequences, from simply feeling defeated to literally giving birth on the pavement.[63] Women who are actually in the hospital often say they are told, 'it will be ages yet' in spite of knowing that the birth is imminent. Others even say they have the urge to push and are told to wait until they are given further instruction by professionals. Again, the clock and the measure and the machine take precedence over the less easily quantifiable female instinct and intuition, and the need for patriarchal control of the powerful process of creating new life pushes aside women's trust and confidence in their own bodies.

# Give birth like an adult

If I could have known all this when I stood looking at my newly pregnant reflection a decade ago, what could I have done? If I had known that so much of my fear and doubt came from assumptions and misguided beliefs that I had picked up and learned through a lifetime in the bubble of my own personal culture, with its long, long history of control and ownership of women's bodies, its fear of their reproductive powers, its total lack of understanding of their anatomy and its mistrust in their ability to function without being heroically rescued, what could I have done? And if I'd known I was about to enter into a maternity care system that was not only built on this bedrock of female dysfunction and pathology but now had the more modern layers of faith-in-the-machine and fear of litigation added in for good measure, what could I have done? If we are to 'give birth like a feminist,' we probably need to consider this question.

The answer, I think, is in awareness – in being what is now sometimes described as 'woke'. Fear, which some people say is an acronym for false evidence appearing real, is very disempowering – we risk becoming rabbits in the headlights, passive at just the moment that action is needed. And as anyone who has ever been in therapy will tell you, at least 50 per cent of the process of change is acknowledging that change is needed. When I set up the Positive Birth Movement, I had been working as a dramatherapist for several years – it's a kind of psychotherapy that uses creativity and story to help people find form for their feelings. In my deep sense of frustration about what was happening to women in childbirth, I turned to what I had learned as a therapist and in my own experiences of being in therapy – that the only thing you really have the power to change is yourself. However, when you start to change yourself – the roles you play, the patterns you habitually fall into – something interesting happens: those around you find that they have to respond to this 'new you' in a different way. And, suddenly, they have to change too. To pick a couple of simple examples, an overly helpful person needs someone who is often seeking their help – and vice versa. A persistent complainer needs someone who is happy to stand and listen to their grievances – and vice versa. Looking at the maternity care system, I thought – this is impossible! How can we ever change this huge sprawling beast?! But when I applied that simple principle I had learned in the world of therapy, it became clear. Rather than try to change the system, why not change the women who enter into the system. What if women turned up at the hospital with an entirely different mindset? With confidence in their bodies, high expectations for their birth experience, knowledge about their choices, and an awareness of their human rights? Wouldn't the 'system' then have to change to accommodate them?

Also helpful to me in my thinking was the branch of psychotherapy known as transactional analysis.* Put very simply, this way of looking at human interactions divides us up into three main 'ego states': Adult, Parent, and Child. In every exchange, we choose to play one of these roles, and the role the other person chooses to play will combine with our own choice and needs to create either a positive or negative experience. So, for example, we might take the Parent role with our partner, telling them, 'Why don't you wash up more often?' and they might respond in Child, 'I don't feel very well, why are you always picking on me?' Or we might be at work and find that we slip into Child role in a meeting, 'Oh, I'm so hopeless, I just can't complete things on time!' while our colleague slips into Parent: 'I'm really disappointed in your lack of commitment.' Again, these states are co-dependent, and one encourages and makes space for the other. They are not always negative, but it's usually better for all of us (providing we actually are adults!) to be in the Adult state. In Adult, we may say, 'I'd really appreciate it if you would do this

---

*    For more on TA see *Games People Play* by Eric Berne and *I'm OK, You're OK* by Thomas A. Harris.

washing up, it's your turn today' or 'I don't have the full report just yet, but I do have a great draft to discuss with you.' And by taking the Adult role, we often nudge others in the transaction to take up the Adult role, too.

At the moment, the maternity care system could really do with some intensive work with a transactional analysis specialist. So often, care providers are trapped in the Parent role, by turns controlling and nurturing, and pregnant women take the role of Child in the transaction, seeking direction and permission, and also, at times, rebelling. Women are kept in the Child state by the constant cultural reinforcement that their bodies don't work without help, in other words, they are dependent, helpless, needy, and powerless, just like children often are. Women often *feel* infantilised by their birth experience, being told they are a 'good girl,' to 'hop up on the bed,' and not being properly informed or consulted about their choices. They can feel they are 'told off' by their care providers, or that they cannot ask questions, or that they must 'do as they are told'. The labour ward can feel a bit like 'back to school'. Transactional analysis teaches us that there *is* something we can do about this – and that's a particularly vital message for somebody persistently stuck in Child, a role that can be inherently helpless. What is needed, is for women in maternity care situations to move into the role of Adult. In doing so, we take away the opportunities for the 'system' to play the role of Parent, and, instead, encourage care providers to take the role of Adult too. This change could transform maternity care, and all it requires is for women to reject the narrative that has been constructed, in which we are weak, dependent, fragile and in need of rescue. As I stood, pregnant in front of my mirror, I had already slipped into Child mode: 'How am I going to give birth? It's impossible. I'm scared. I don't want to!' If only I had been more aware of how this was not truly fact, but simply fears I had learned from my culture, I might have said to my reflection: 'I'm an adult, I'm a woman, I'm strong and I can do this.' And that's a game changer.

# Chapter 6
# Birth and Culture: 'Fish can't see water'

*Feminine bodily existence is an inhibited intentionality, which simultaneously reaches toward a projected end with an 'I can' and withholds its full bodily commitment to that end in a self-imposed 'I cannot'.*

Iris Marion Young, 'Throwing Like a Girl'[1]

I'd always reconciled myself to the fact that I would live my entire life many degrees of separation away from Kim Kardashian's bottom, but I'm delighted to tell you that, as of November 2014, all that changed. Depending on whether or not you follow Kim – and her bottom – you may or may not remember that images of her oiled derriere 'broke the internet' when she posed for the cover of *Paper* magazine. My own involvement in the story came when, by sheer coincidence, I was banned from Facebook at the exact same moment for sharing a photo of a woman having a water birth. The image was taken from behind and you could see the baby beginning to emerge. In other words, it was another rear view of a bottom.

This wasn't my first transgression. Just under a year previously I'd been banned for sharing two birth images, again via the Positive Birth Movement social media pages, one of which showed a dimly lit naked woman in profile, kneeling on a bed to give birth, and the other showed a mother's hands catching her own baby as it emerged under water in a pool. For this I'd been given a 48-hour ban, but for my second offence of the birthing bottom, they banned me for a week and demanded I send a copy of my passport to identify myself. It's important to add that images normally only get removed because somebody reports them, so we can see this as a censorship of the images by wider society – it's not just a 'Facebook' problem.

## A tale of two bottoms

As I sat feeling outraged and scrolling through Twitter for comfort, I couldn't help noticing that every second tweet was about Kim's naked and uncensored backside and the irony of my situation began to become clear. With a picture of Kim's bottom and the birthing bottom side by side, I tweeted, 'How come some bums are OK and some bums are not? I'm confused Facebook,' adding in a second tweet, 'Some nudity approved, some gets you banned.' The tweets sparked media coverage around the world, perhaps not quite the quantity needed to 'break the internet,' but enough to start a conversation about how we view women's bodies and how some seem to meet with more approval than others. In the ensuing debate, I felt it important that it did not become a criticism of Kim, or her decision to show off her body, thereby descending into another polarised 'mummy war'. Women should feel free to express pride in their bodies and confidence in their naked flesh, however they see fit. Instead I wanted to turn the spotlight on why these particular images of women's bodies in labour were considered unacceptable, and in need of censorship.

The first thing to note about all three of the images that got me banned is that they are not the kind of birth images we are most used to seeing. If you stop people in the street and ask them to picture a woman in labour and then describe her, you'll get some fairly standard themes – 'on a bed,' 'on her back,' 'screaming,' 'swearing at her husband,' 'in a hospital gown,' 'surrounded by doctors,' 'looking deranged with pain,' and so on. These images were different. They showed the female body in powerful action: not passively inviting the approval or judgement of another's gaze, but in the midst of actually *doing* something incredible. Composed, vital and beautiful, as opposed to 'in distress,' the women in the photos are not 'being delivered,' but catching their babies themselves. As I wrote in the *Guardian* at the time of the first ban, 'The images challenge everything many people wrongly assume to be true about childbirth and show the female body naked, shameless, real, capable, useful, active, empowered. This is why women need to see these images; and this is why they are censored.'[2]

Or, to quote T.S. Eliot, 'Human kind cannot bear very much reality,'[3] and this certainly seems to be true when it comes to the depiction of women and their bodies. Our menstrual blood on the tampon ads is blue. Recently one or two models have broken taboos by being photographed with leg hair – and received rape and death threats.[4] Instagram has famously removed images of women with pubic hair protruding from their knickers, of vaginal discharge, and of period-stained undies.[5] Celebrity nipples often pass the censors, but breastfeeding women are still getting social media bans,[6] in spite of policies that say their images are welcome. And, of course, nursing mums are still being told to 'cover up'[7] in real life, too.[8] Against this cultural backdrop, you can see why a birthing bottom might cause alarm – as one person said to me on social media at the time, 'It's disgusting – it's not right for kids to see that.'

As a mother of three – and two are girls – I would beg to differ. I would far rather my children grew up with the confidence in their skin that comes from knowing the truth about the capabilities of their amazing bodies, than the inadequacy that stems from not only the objectification of women but also the projection of a totally unreal version of womanhood – airbrushed, passive and fake – that so many of us have been taught to aspire to. Why spend a lifetime feeling inadequate because we can never be that hairless, streamlined, contoured 'princess'? Our blood really isn't blue – nor should we want it to be.

Women's lack of confidence in the birth room might be traced back through this cultural maze. We grow up conditioned to distance ourselves from the reality of our bodies: our fat, our hair, our discharge, our sweat, our blood. With many women being taught that their periods are shameful, dirty and a 'curse,' we can see the seeds of female bodily anxiety being planted early. Germaine Greer famously said, 'If you think you are emancipated, you might consider the idea of tasting your own menstrual blood – if it makes you sick, you've got a long way to go, baby,'[9] and over 40 years later, this quote still has the power to shock. Tasting our period blood seems extreme in a world where we very often try not to even look at it, keeping it hidden from ourselves and others. And again, this shame becomes intergenerational, part of the 'broken chain of wisdom' – it's hard to teach your daughter body confidence and period positivity when the opposite has been so deeply ingrained in you personally, and when negative messages about femaleness continue to pervade our wider culture.

> *Labor is totally incongruent with the myths of delicate,*
> *weak femininity.*
> *The laboring body is thus almost an oxymoron:*
> *the 'feminine body' in the highest sense (birthing,*
> *accomplishing the task of femininity, revealing the*
> *'mysterious essence' of women), but also a strong,*
> *active, creative body, capable of enduring and*
> *recovering from the splitting of its flesh. This is what*
> *makes it dangerous, prone to domestication and*
> *control.*
>
> Sara Cohen Shabot[10]

# Bare reality

Like periods, birth is often seen as something dysfunctional or 'gross'. As we approach it as women, this becomes part of our fear – we don't wish to be too 'real,' too 'exposed,' too 'loud' or too 'out of control'. Some women may not wish to have the experience of vaginal birth at all due to an aversion to the leaky, bloody, noisy nature of it all. 'I don't see any reason to give birth like a cow in this day and age when there are more civilised means available,' one woman told researchers enquiring into the motivations of women who choose caesareans in 2011.[11] Reasons for caesarean choice are complex, but the desire to keep hold of what is perceived as 'control' or 'dignity' is often a factor. The epidural, too, offers a more 'calm' and 'controlled' environment on the labour ward – for both women and their care providers too – with much less of the loud, guttural or animalistic noises that women in the throes of labour may make, and which are often another element of birth that women fear.

We must be quiet, and we must also be hairless. The removal of leg, armpit and pubic hair is a well-covered area of feminist discussion, with nobody quite sure why we are all still doing it. Some feel the trend, particularly for pube removal, originates in pornography; others speculate it began in earnest in the seventies out of an unconscious desire to infantilise women at a time they were campaigning loudly for equal rights. Hairless certainly indicates 'pre-pubescent,' 'little girl,' which does make you wonder why, for the last half-century or so, there's been a bit of an obsession with pubes in the birth room, a place where women are so often treated like children. Women no longer have routine pubic shaves before birth – in the UK at least, although it still happens in many other countries including Italy, India, Bulgaria, Greece, Romania, Kenya, France, Spain and Brazil – but forums and online articles are buzzing with advice on how to prepare yourself 'down there'. 'Many women will take it upon themselves to remove all of their hair before labour,' UK midwife Katy Blundell told me. 'And the ones that haven't had time often won't stop apologising – although as midwives we really don't care either way!' In fact, there is good evidence that pubic hair has a value in birth (as it does at all other times) – the hair itself provides protection from infection, added to which depilation before birth can also cause microscopic open wounds, an extra infection risk.[12] How ironic that, 40 years ago or so, a UK woman would have routinely got a non-evidence-based shave (very often without proper consent either), but now that this practice is no longer allowed or recommended, women are anxiously removing their own pubes anyway – out of either fashion or concern for their care providers' sensibilities? Tammy Wynette was right, sometimes it really *is* hard to be a woman.

As well as getting their pubes in order, being 'calm' and 'serene' in birth is something women often aspire to, and, for those who want to avoid epidural as a means to this end, hypnobirthing has stepped forward with a solution, offering women the chance to learn how to 'breathe their baby out'. Hypnosis for childbirth itself is a brilliant tool which many women find fantastically helpful, so I'm not trying to critique the technique itself, but rather the way that, because of our cultural fear of birth, it can be misappropriated as a certain way to give birth – 'neat' and 'regulated' – and for some, another test that you can fail. Are you 'doing hypnobirthing right' if you are thrashing around, yelping, howling, crying and begging for an epidural? This might be just a passing phase, probably 'transition,' the moment of full dilation when many women do decide that they want to give up, but if you're hypnobirthing, you might not have expected to be this out of control. Women who are 'calm' in labour are also often praised, 'Isn't she doing well, you would hardly know she was dilating would you?' and those who are 'losing it' might find that they raise concerns that they are 'not coping,' or are even told to 'shhhhh' or to 'try the epidural' – which of course has the side-effect of a much quieter labour ward. And yet giving birth is not always a tidy, linear experience. Just like running a marathon, we may have times when we feel we are hitting our stride and others when we doubt whether we can continue. I like the idea of birth as a 'heroine's journey'. If you're not familiar with this idea, it's sometimes called the 'monomyth,'* and it's basically a template or pattern that many stories follow – think *Star Wars*, the *Hunger Games*, the *Lion King*, *Harry Potter*, *Lord of the Rings*, *The Wizard of Oz*, the *Odyssey* and so many more. The pattern goes something like this: the hero, who starts in a normal situation, gets a call to adventure, is filled with doubt, then sets off on a journey that includes: meeting a mentor, fighting off enemies, a 'road of trials,' descent into an underworld, encountering the goddess, a reward, and finally a kind of resurrection

---

\*     For more on the monomyth see Joseph Campbell's, *The Hero with a Thousand Faces*

or rebirth, returning with the prize or elixir back to the 'real world,' but ultimately transformed by the experience. The monomyth is said to be based on the unconscious patterns that reoccur constantly in myths and stories, but if those patterns themselves didn't originate in the path every woman treads to bring new life into the world, I'll eat my light sabre.

Every woman who has a baby, however that baby is ultimately born, treads this path of the heroine, and yet it's not always perceived that way. By making real women's experiences and stories so immediately accessible, social media is playing a big role in challenging this, and showing women the reality of childbirth in a world in which they have become largely removed from it. Since my Facebook bans back in 2013 and 2014, Facebook and Instagram have been repeatedly pressurised to allow more 'real' images of women and have softened their approach to censoring birth. Although it still happens, there are now more inclusive standards in place. In 2018, Instagram publicly updated their policy on birth images,[13] following a petition that gained over 20,000 signatures. 'We believe (the new policy) better categorises birthing images as educational and celebratory,' they said, and this represented a real step forwards. And, of course, it's not all about the 'graphic' pictures of babies actually emerging, although these do so much to break down misperceptions. Women also just want to see what women who are in labour or who have just had babies 'look like,' as I discovered in 2015, when I shared an article on the Positive Birth Movement Facebook page about the photographer Jenny Lewis's latest project, 'One Day Young'.[14] Lewis took a series of beautiful photographs of women, the day after childbirth, because she wanted to 'tell a story about the strength and resilience of women, post-childbirth,' that she felt, 'goes largely unacknowledged in today's world'. Having had two good births herself, she felt the need to 'dilute the fear surrounding birth'. 'All I ever heard about was epidurals and caesareans and pain and fear – there was no positive information.'[15] Lewis's work was perfect in its own right, but when I shared it on social media, something truly wonderful happened. Suddenly and spontaneously, other new mothers started sharing their own images of themselves in the first minutes or hours of their babies' lives, because they too felt passionately that they wished to 'dilute the fear'.

# #birthjusthappened

In trying to come up with a hashtag for women's post-birth images and stories, I searched for an idea that summed up both the fact that they had just given birth, and also that it wasn't anything dreadful – an everyday occurrence not an illness or an operation. Into my mind popped #birthjusthappened, and over the next few days, hundreds of women sent in images of their glowing and triumphant faces in the wake of all kinds of births that had 'just happened'. Again, there was wide media coverage, with headlines like, 'The photos changing the way we see labour'[16] and 'Post birth selfies are exactly what women need.'[17] The women who participated by sending in their pics spoke repeatedly about wishing to challenge cultural misconceptions of childbirth and help other women to be less afraid. Beki Kemp, from Somerset in the UK, who shared an image of herself after her second baby was born in water, told me at the time that 'Birth is portrayed as "the most painful and unpredictable event of your life". It was only after my first birth that I realised how much the way birth is talked about had affected me. I just thought the horror stories were the norm.' Another who shared an image, Luella Shapiro from Wisconsin, said, 'I'd like women to see that it's not all horror stories and emergencies. It's beautiful and intense and emotional all at once. I think these pictures are so helpful to see because they contradict the idea that women are powerless, sick, drugged, or otherwise weak and passive during birth. They show that birth can be something powerful and strong and beautiful, and that can give pregnant women – especially first-timers – confidence going forward into their own births.'

The appetite for this new narrative around childbirth is massive. Women want to soak up these positive stories, messages and images, as if self-administering the antidote to decades or more of negativity and fear. In our image-driven age, a picture can paint a thousand words. At the time of #birthjusthappened I spoke to pregnant women about the images. 'I was dreading giving birth in two weeks' time,' one of them told me. 'But now I'm amazed to say I'm looking forward to it – I feel incredibly excited after seeing these pictures,' while another commented, 'You can really feel the power in these photos. This is the kind of birth I didn't know existed, but now really want.' Women are often warned about 'the reality of childbirth,' but social media is offering them an opportunity to have an uncensored discussion about this – with films and images to illustrate their point – and the secret that many of them seem to be sharing is this: *It's not that bad, and you can do it.*

# #birthundisturbed

This was the message that Natalie Lennard wanted to share when, in 2017, she departed from her usual work as the highly regarded 'surreal fashion' photographer 'Miss Aniela,' and began the project Birth Undisturbed.[18] The images were recreations of famous moments and ideas from the history of birth, from Grantly Dick-Read's 'Whitechapel Woman' who famously told him, 'It didn't hurt. It wasn't meant to, was it, doctor?'[19] to the Queen giving birth at home to Prince Edward, to the birth of Jesus depicted – not in the manger afterwards as we normally see him – but graphically emerging into Mary's bloody hands. Other shots in the series depicted concepts such as the 'salle sauvage' – the idea of a particular primal space for birth, a 'primitive room,' originated by obstetrician Michel Odent; another shows the 'Fetal Ejection Reflex' in action as a woman gives birth on her doorstep on her way to the hospital. Just as I experienced with #birthjusthappened, Lennard wanted to challenge the usual cultural portrayal of birth. 'I'd been shooting fashion models for years, and seeing pictures of women looking beautiful and sexy and young and feminine, and all these things, but never really quite powerful,' she told me. 'That is what this series is all about. That's what I want to put out there, this new imagery showing the whole wonder and the emotions and textures of childbirth. I think that we're starved of images like this.' As with #birthjusthappened, the feedback from women about Natalie's images seems to support the idea that they are genuinely nourishing to a generation of women who are craving positive birth messages. One woman commented on Lennard's Instagram,[20] 'I thought of your model mother's powerful expressions while I was in active labour, which was hugely empowering. Because of your work I went from dreading labour as something to be endured, to anticipating it as what would likely be the most powerful and transformative experience of my life, which is exactly what it was.' Another said, 'Your images have illuminated the fact that childbirth isn't to be feared, which is definitely not the impression I had most of my life. Can't really express how powerful that is. I feel like because of people like you, there is a sort of birth revolution going on, and it's fucking magical.'

Social media is helping to revolutionise women's postnatal experiences, too. The reaction to Kate Middleton's body shape when she left hospital just a day after giving birth to Prince George in 2013 was pretty astonishing, with some media outlets baffled about how she 'still has a baby bump'. Experts were called in to explain to journalists how the female form doesn't ping back to the way it was before right away (or possibly ever), even if you are a duchess, and the ensuing newspaper articles showed just how embarrassingly little we know about postpartum bodies. Instagram and Facebook have the answer to this too though, with more and more women – including some celebrities – sharing pictures of their 'post-baby bodies,' including their 'bumps' in the time after birth, their stretch marks, their caesarean scars and their large underwear and pads under hashtags like #takebackpostpartum and #stopcensoringmotherhood. All of this social media activity around birth feels like part of the fourth wave of feminism, defined predominantly by technology and sometimes called 'hashtag feminism' – think #metoo, #everydaysexism, #nomorepage3 and so many more campaigns in which women have used social media to challenge the status quo. The power of the internet to shake up thinking and mobilise grassroots action is proving to be transformational in so many areas of women's lives, and in birth the current wave of activism feels fresh, vibrant and long overdue. Alongside this youthful and energetic phenomenon, however, a dinosaur continues to lumber, one that we can only hope is on its last legs – the ancient and scaly beast known as 'One Born Every Minute'.

## One born every minute

It's frustrating how the TV series *One Born Every Minute* (OBEM) – and if you're not in the UK or the USA where it is aired, you probably have a similar fly-on-the-wall labour ward docu-drama that follows different couples as they arrive at the hospital to have their baby – has become engrained in the fabric of our television lives and, for so many women, a template of 'what birth is like'. And yet the births on the programme, except in the rarest cases, portray women on beds, on their backs, at the mercy of both the forces of nature and of the decisions of their care providers. Of course, this is a television programme, and it needs to hold our attention – so it could be argued that this is a fair excuse for birth being painted as a dramatic, fast-paced emergency. Long, slow, dimly lit and uneventful labours might be better for women, but they probably wouldn't make such compelling viewing. Added to this, the programme makers probably find it easier to film medicalised births, which often take place on a hospital bed – perfect for camera angles as well as obstetricians, perhaps. Births will also be in daytime hours, and easier to work into a busy filming schedule, if they are induced. It might also be possible that a woman who has done their homework on birth physiology would be less likely to agree to take part in the programme – for being observed and filmed could potentially hamper the natural progress of labour – making it more likely that those who do consent to be on the programme are less aware of how to promote normal birth for themselves, and probably more willing to comply with hospital norms and protocols.

All of these and more are great excuses for the portrayal of birth on *OBEM*, but the bottom line is this – the programme has a powerful influence on women and their partners, and therefore arguably has a social responsibility to start including more information about women's options and rights in the birth room. Many midwives and birth workers will admit to watching *OBEM* through the gaps between their fingers, cringing at the portrayal of their profession. 'I can't watch it any more, it's bad for my blood pressure,' one told me, while another added, 'I cannot bear to watch the way so many opportunities for a straightforward woman-centred birth experience are missed.' If you follow the Twitter feed for the programme, you can also see many examples of pregnant women being affected by it. 'Watching old episodes of *One Born Every Minute* to mentally prepare myself for torture. I am terrified even though I know what to expect,' tweeted @laurastonex. 'Watching *One Born Every Minute* – probably shouldn't though, knowing that's going to be me in a week's time (anxious face),' said @wldxhrt. There is also plenty of humour about how horrible birth appears to be, with @goggleboxAU describing it as 'the contraception we didn't know we needed'.

*OBEM*, and docu-dramas like it, are damaging to women. By presenting birth in this way, we are normalising and perpetuating a culture where having a baby is viewed as a medical emergency in which women have little or no voice. This has a direct knock-on effect on women's birth expectations, and, in turn, their behaviour, fear levels, trust in their bodies and sense of autonomy in the birth room itself. But the programme isn't out on a limb, it's part of a long history of the depiction of birth on screen as a dysfunctional crisis from which women must be urgently rescued. Think of almost any birth you have ever seen on film and you will have a mix of similar elements: a rush to the hospital, a bed, doctors taking charge, a helpless sweaty woman on her back, everyone yelling, 'Push!' And most often, immediate cutting of the cord (if there even is a cord – Rachel's baby in *Friends* is one example of a baby that comes out already detached!), no skin-to-skin contact with the baby, and never a placenta in sight. In an attempt to challenge this, US childbirth educator Vicki Elson created a film called, *Labouring Under an Illusion: Mass Media Childbirth vs The Real Thing*[21] in 2009, juxtaposing births on TV with real footage of labouring women, sometimes to humorous effect, but with a serious point to make about just how unrealistic birth on TV can be. One of the best things a twenty-first-century pregnant woman can do is seek out films like Elson's and other online birth movies, that show home birth, water birth, upright birth – indeed any kind of birth where the woman is queen of the room, in control and in her power.

And the worst thing she can probably do is watch *One Born Every Minute* – unless she views it simply as a way to learn more about what hospital birth can be like if you don't know your options. If you think I'm being harsh on the nation's favourite night in, you might be interested to know that several academics have examined the programme in detail and raised similar concerns. Professor of Psychosocial Theory at Birkbeck, Lisa Baraitser, and Sociology Professor Imogen Tyler, wrote a paper in 2013[22] in *Studies in the Maternal* that concluded that *OBEM*, like many other childbirth TV shows, portrays women as 'largely passive subjects,' and that the programme encourages a very limited view of the possibilities for birth 'outside of dominant systems of control and surveillance that characterise obstetric practices in the Global North'. On top of this, *OBEM* creates fear, that 'feeds into and reproduces ideas of birth as a "crisis" which needs to be managed to a successful conclusion by medical experts'.

Researcher Julie Roberts leads a Wellcome Trust-funded project called Televising Childbirth, an interdisciplinary group of researchers at the University of Nottingham who have been exploring the ways in which birth is represented on television and how this might affect women's experiences. As part of this they have conducted a quantitative 'content analysis' of *One Born Every Minute*,[23] finding that not only does the programme over-represent white, heterosexual couples, it also shows a 'medicalisation of birth through the routinisation of supposedly minor birth interventions, and the absence of the representation of women's choice over such interventions'. Over the two series they studied, they found that no home births were represented, and any birth in a midwife-led unit was not made clear, potentially leading to the impression, especially to the lay viewer, that all births took place in an obstetric setting. 90 per cent of women in the final 'pushing' stages of labour were shown on their backs, 98 per cent of births included pain relief, and 77 per cent featured interventions – all of this contributes to what the researchers neatly describe as the programme's capacity to 'make the commonplace appear normal' – in other words, this may happen all the time in labour wards up and down the land, but presenting it to us on our screens in this way without question, encourages us to accept it as 'the way birth is'.

The 'Televising Childbirth' team also highlight the striking lack of information that is given to labouring women on *OBEM* about their options and choices. In 91 per cent of birth stories depicting a procedure, for example, the viewer is not shown a discussion about the woman's choice. The researchers acknowledge that this does not necessarily mean that women were not given information or choices, but simply that it wasn't depicted within the programme. However, this in itself is problematic – it effectively sidelines the subject of women's birth choices and keeps any conversation about this vital issue out of the mainstream, and 'potentially positions women as subordinate to the birth process, their bodies and those considered more able to make birth decisions'. Researcher Julie Roberts told me, 'I'm particularly concerned about the lack of explanation for intervention and the absence of discussions with women on camera about the pros, cons and alternative options. I think seeing these conversations happening on mainstream TV would be really positive in terms of promoting and supporting women's autonomy and choices in labour.'

*If you don't know your options, you don't have any.*

Diana Korte[24]

Some researchers have even looked at the conversations that take place between women and midwives on *OBEM* and analysed these interactions to explore how decisions were made. Jackson et al. at the University of York published a paper in 2016 entitled, 'Healthcare professionals' assertions and women's responses during labour: a conversation analytic study of data from *One Born Every Minute*'.[25] Through transcribing and studying 26 conversations, they found that the midwives on *OBEM* frequently used what they term 'assertions,' which affected the sense of actual choice experienced by the women. Midwives on the programme would often say, 'We need to . . . ,' or 'We're going to . . . ,' for example 'We need to put you on a monitor now,' or 'We're just going to break your waters'. The subtext of framing choice in this way, of course, is that it isn't a choice at all. No consent or permission is being sought – rather the proposed course of action is presented as *necessary* or *going to happen*. The use of the word 'We' implies that several people support this decision – rendering the labouring woman more isolated and vulnerable in any objection – and also implies that it's a joint decision and that the woman is somehow already in agreement. The researchers point out that their study of the programme may expose a gap between current policies on shared decision making in maternity care, and what is actually happening at ground level.

It's interesting to see the findings of this research because women often report bitter personal experience of this gap between policy and reality. Often, they highlight dehumanised and out-dated language, including 'delivered' – women give birth, pizzas are delivered, so it was a surprise to see this terminology in the title for another recent birth documentary presented by Emma Willis, *Delivering Babies*. Kati Edwards, a doula whose own home birth was filmed for the one-off BBC documentary *Childbirth: All or Nothing* in 2016, felt that much of the content of *Delivering Babies* was, like the title, yet another missed opportunity to move the conversation forward. 'Had nobody told the programme makers that the use of the word "deliver" is hotly debated in maternity circles? Changing the language we use around birth may seem like a series of subtle distinctions but it's one of the crucial elements needing to happen in order to hand birth back to women before we lose it altogether,' she told me. 'Added to this the programme was filled with examples of care that was not woman-centred: yelling at women to push, telling them it's normal to feel you've been hit by a train after childbirth, and even chit-chatting away and disturbing a woman all the way through what should have been a peaceful home birth. It left me feeling irate!'[26] For most people, though, *Delivering Babies*, like *OBEM*, is heart-warming entertainment, viewed by the majority without objection. Image by image, scene by scene, such shows 'make the commonplace appear normal,' shaping the expectations – and by default, the reality – of everyone who ever has a baby, or is in the room while she does so. Like Kim Kardashian's passive bottom, these versions of birth are considered totally acceptable, while those in which women are active and have agency are rare, censored, or not even given airtime in the first place.

# The gore of childbirth

In the print media, too, birth is sensationalised and stories of drama and danger are always favoured over tales of powerful women nailing it. As I write, a quick search of recent headlines shows the usual suspects – words like 'horror,' 'risk' and 'pain' appear frequently. Having written about birth in the media for several years I know from experience that editors will often pick 'click bait' headlines to draw in readers in this competitive online age. One piece I wrote about fathers suffering PTSD after childbirth, which challenged our cultural acceptance of birth as inherently traumatic and suggested that it didn't have to be this way – for dads, mums, or indeed anyone – was given the headline, 'Men need to better prepare for the gore of childbirth,'[27] which seemed quite a long way from the point I was trying to make. In two and a half years as a weekly columnist for *BestDaily* magazine, editor Abigail Blackburn and I worked as a team to create both content – and matching headlines – to upend the existing narrative about birth and present it from an entirely different, more woman-centred and feminist, angle, but no one was expecting the traffic our approach generated. Our partnership began during Kate Middleton's first pregnancy, when Abigail asked me to write about the media response to the Duchess's rumoured desire for a drug-free hypnobirth. In a short opinion piece, entitled, 'Is Kate being bullied about her birth?,' we took on the media headlines that poured scorn on her plans and undermined her self-confidence, and asked why the world was so keen to mock women like Kate who felt that they could cope with the challenge of a natural labour. The article quickly went viral, and I was soon hired to write a weekly column. 'We were the only mainstream publication at the time to defend Kate's choices,' Abigail said. 'That one article transformed a small website launch into a record-breaking overnight success at Hearst Magazines, delivering so much traffic I received calls from IT asking me if I'd broken the system. What was most gratifying was seeing comments from readers on social media, who were especially excited that our women-centred angles were being published in a well-known and mainstream brand like Best. That meant so much to people that they would return in droves week after week, just to see what headline we would say next, and we continued to break traffic records. It just went to show that there has been a silent majority who wanted to be spoken for and about with positivity, encouragement and respect for their birth choices, even if they were first-time mothers.'

# WHAT IS POSITIVE BIRTH?

The following is from www.positivebirthmovement.org. The Positive Birth Movement believes that every woman deserves a positive birth. But what does this mean?
Here's how we define it:

- Women are where they want to be
- Choices are informed by reality not fear
- Women are listened to and treated with respect and dignity
- Mothers are empowered and enriched
- Memories are warm and proud

A positive birth means a birth in which a woman feels she has freedom of choice, access to accurate information, and that she is in control, powerful and respected. A birth that she approaches, perhaps with some trepidation, but without fear or dread, and later remembers with warmth and pride.

A positive birth does not have to be 'natural' or 'drug free' – it simply has to be informed from a place of positivity as opposed to fear. The Positive Birth Movement is woman-centred and as such respects a woman's right to choose where and how she has her baby.

You can birth with positivity in hospital or at home, with or without medical intervention. You can have a positive caesarean, or a positive home water birth. Positive Birth is about approaching birth realistically, having genuine choice, and feeling empowered by your experience.

The Positive Birth Movement believes that communication is the key to shaking up birth. By coming together, in real life and online, and sharing experiences, feelings, knowledge and wisdom, women can take back childbirth.

Saying you want a natural birth, or a home birth, is going to make waves, whether you are Kate, Meghan, or just plain old you having a lemonade in your local. I can still remember how one of the old boys at the bar in my nearest pub laughed his head off at me when I said I didn't think I wanted an epidural. 'You'll soon change your tune, love!' he guffawed – just 'banter,' of course, but as any woman reading this will know, a lifetime of 'banter' can have a slow-drip effect, gradually wearing us thin. In this case, I felt a little tiny wave of self-doubt and embarrassment in the wake of his comments, and he was left feeling like the pub wit. But as women, having our choices judged is part of the fabric of our lives – I might have equally expected scrutiny had I said I was having a planned caesarean – in fact, it's hard to think of a choice I could have made that would *not* have been subject to some kind of analysis. Postnatally, too, there is often debate about what birth stories women should or should not share. Women who had positive experiences can be accused of 'showing off' or 'shaming' other women if they speak about their births, but likewise, women who had difficult or traumatic experiences can be accused of filling other women with fear and even causing tokophobia. Whether your birth plans are still on the drawing board or in pieces on the floor, be prepared to come under fire if you share them. Ever since my beginnings at *BestDaily*, I've always had a soft spot for Kate Middleton, and I'm reminded of how, as she's stood on the steps of the Lindo Wing, she's been simultaneously accused of still having a bump and looking like she *has* just had a baby, and appearing too glamourous and fit and looking like she *hasn't* just had a baby. Like the rest of us, it seems, Kate is damned either way.

Partners can also find that discussing their thoughts about birth or retelling their experiences is complex terrain. It's becoming more acceptable for men to share their feelings about becoming fathers, with trails being blazed by celebrities like Russell Brand, who described his partner Laura giving birth in 2017 in metaphysical terms, 'she becomes yet more holy, inhibitions exhaled, a sense of immersion and self-realisation . . . "These women know what they are doing," I think,'[28] or The Rock, who posted on Instagram in 2018, 'If you really want to understand the most powerful and primal moment life will ever offer, watch your child being born.'[29] In general, though, to talk about childbirth like Brand – 'a sense of being held, guided, carried . . . by the pathway already walked by all of our ancestors' – is unusual, and you're more likely to get positive feedback if you take the Robbie Williams line – he described it as, 'watching my favourite pub burn down,' and Emma Thompson then wrote it in as one of her character's lines in *Bridget Jones's Baby*.[30] 'Watching my favourite pub burn down': this potentially tells you more about why birth is a feminist issue in six words than this book will do in ninety thousand. The woman is entirely dehumanised and objectified, becoming not a person but a place – an entertainment location built to serve the needs of her man, and childbirth will completely destroy this. Oh, and P.S, that's *funny* – funny enough for a blockbuster movie. Maybe I'm overreacting. Perhaps it was just 'banter'.

# #soproud: celebrating new mothers

Partners are not exempt from the so-called birth wars. The footballer Harry Kane ran into hot water in 2018 when he tweeted that he was 'so proud' that his wife had given birth without pain relief. Immediately he faced a barrage of criticism, with headlines proclaiming that he had 'turned childbirth into a competitive sport' and 'put his golden boot in it,' adding, somewhat inevitably, that, 'no one cares how you give birth as long as the baby is safely delivered'.[31] Unwittingly, Kane had tapped into the dark seam of anger and hurt that runs under the surface of the childbirth conversation, and discovered just how highly charged any comment about birth choices can be. After twenty-four hours of being savaged on Twitter, he issued an apology, and I found myself feeling irked on his behalf – why should we not be able to say we are proud of someone for doing something that others have chosen not to do, or were not able to do? And where do we draw the line, if this is to be the ruling? Can a partner not say they are 'so proud' of their wife for their bravery during a caesarean, or for giving birth at home, or for knowing that the time was right to take the epidural? Must we all censor not just our birth stories, but our emotions about them too? Surely every woman who gives birth is a hero, no matter what choices she makes or how it pans out for her, and their partners should be free to be as proud as they like. These feelings of frustration led to another viral hashtag campaign on the Positive Birth Movement, #soproud, where women and their partners shared their birth images and stories and their reasons for being proud. These reasons were many and varied – from birth without drugs to twin caesarean and even to stories of baby loss – but one clear theme emerged: women appreciated a space where they could talk freely about these experiences and give themselves praise for the power and strength they had found in themselves. This space is currently missing in our society.

In other cultures, and in other times in history, the new mother would have been cared for and celebrated, but often, this could not be further from the truth in the twenty-first-century Western world. Women are quickly discharged from hospital, often with little or no support in place at home, and left to get on with it. Sometimes the proposed solution is that we go back to a longer postnatal stay in hospital, but this doesn't really address the underlying problem of attitudes to the woman who has just given birth – just as we seem to have lost the capacity to treat labouring women like goddesses, so too have we become unable to worship, venerate, elevate and cherish women postnatally. In other cultures, there is often a mandatory period of rest for new mothers, where visitors are limited or kept away, special nourishing foods are prepared, and the mother is massaged, sung to, bathed, anointed with oils or showered with gifts. In Tanzania, women are not expected to do anything other than eat, sleep and care for their baby for the first four months, and when they go anywhere, people call out 'Nawore mfee!' ('She has just given birth'), signifying that she must be respected and given priority. In China, new mothers follow Zuo Yuezi ('sitting the month'), resting in bed at the home of their mother-in-law or mother for thirty days, keeping very warm, and eating special 'hot' foods, according to the principles of yin and yang.[32] Western women may not appreciate mandatory rest at the mother-in-law's, but they might like *kraamzorg,* a standard part of the state-funded maternity care system in the Netherlands, providing a home helper or *kraamverzorgster* for at least eight hours a day, for eight days postpartum. The *kraamverzorgster* supports the mother, helping her to learn to look after her newborn, get breastfeeding established, and cleaning her house and making food for her.

# CELEBRATING YOURSELF POSTNATALLY

If you've just given birth, no matter how your baby made their entrance (or exit!), you have just done something amazing. However, once the first few days are over and the bunches of flowers begin to wilt, you may still feel that you need more focus, not on the baby, but on you personally, what you just experienced, and how you are now feeling. You may also feel a pressure to carry on as you were before the birth, focusing on not only work and practical tasks but also on 'getting your body back'. Take this pressure off, and pause. As you recover from birth, the following suggestions may help you to feel nourished and celebrated.

## Tell or write your story

It can be hard to find ears to listen to your birth story – at least not the detailed version. But whether your experience was positive or traumatic, it can be so important for someone to hear it. If you did have a traumatic birth then it can help to go over what happened with your midwife, and if you request this, they may have a formal 'birth reflections' service where they can go over your notes with you and explain what happened. You may also find groups on social media where you can discuss your birth experience. And no matter what kind of birth you had, it's great to write your story down in as much detail as you can remember.

## Bonding with your baby vs. 'self-care'

These two ideas are often sold as separate. In the first few days or weeks, you might be told that you should leave your baby with someone else to get some rest or 'me time'. You might love this, but you may also not feel ready to be parted from your newborn, and this is OK too. Activities like a warm bath together or lying in bed 'skin to skin' can be nurturing for both you and your baby simultaneously. Then, when you are ready, it might also be good to have some time to yourself to do whatever makes you feel good, whether that's exercise, work or a glass of wine with a friend.

## Your post-baby body is normal

Just as many of us have not seen childbirth in 'real life,' we're pretty in the dark about post-baby bodies too. It can be a shock when your glorious, firm and frankly quite sexy bump, suddenly looks more like a deflated balloon. Know that this is normal, and seek out images on social media under hashtags like #takebackpostpartum or #thisispostpartum to reassure you. Know too that most women have mixed feelings about their postnatal form – in awe of what their body has achieved on the one hand and slightly miffed by the stretch marks on the other. Documenting your body with photos – whether or not you choose to share them – is one way that women have taken ownership of this phase. And it is a phase.

## Nurturing food

Before your baby arrives, plan for the postpartum time to be filled with nourishing, healthy food, and with food you love. These might not be the same. That's OK. Make sure you get plenty of nutritious meals stacked in your freezer and on order from your grocery delivery. Line yourself up some treats, too. Think of this time like a holiday where you indulge yourself and celebrate. Keep your dressing gown on if you can for the first couple of weeks, and eat posh ice cream out of the tub and carrot sticks in equal measure (but not together).

## Honour your feelings

Many women struggle with their emotions in the first year of motherhood. This can come in waves or feel worse at particular times, for example when your milk comes in, or when your partner returns to work or your mum or other support leaves. It's totally normal to feel like you are on an emotional rollercoaster at times. However, if these feelings persist, you may be one of the 10 per cent of women who are affected by postnatal depression (PND), or, if you had a traumatic birth, you may be suffering from PTSD. There are other more complex postnatal mental health issues, too, such as postpartum psychosis. For information and support organisations a good place to start is https://www.mind.org.uk/information-support/types-of-mental-health-problems/postnatal-depression-and-perinatal-mental-health/

In the UK and many other countries such as the USA, where maternity leave is just six weeks long, postnatal care that nurtures and cares for the mother is a long way from our reality. We can see this as part of a continuum in which women's issues are sidelined and the entire journey to motherhood is treated as a medical condition rather than a rite of passage. Once the 'healthy baby' has been achieved, there is the cursory postnatal health check, apart from which the woman seems to be unimportant, only held up for praise if she 'gets her body back' and becomes productive again, either by returning to work and/or returning to being and looking sexual. There is a lack of support or funding for women with postnatal mental health issues, many of which have their roots in the birth experience. There are very few spaces for traumatised women to tell their stories; likewise, there are very few spaces, rituals or opportunities to celebrate women's achievement of bringing new life into the world. Motherhood itself is not seen to be a particularly valued task, and many social and political policies encourage new mums to delegate the task of childcare to trained helpers so that they can return to the workplace. Once there, the cost of nursery can sometimes mean they barely break even, but many consider this to be a worthwhile swap in a world where, left alone with a baby, they feel undervalued and isolated. As one woman described it to me, many new mothers live in 'solitary confinement'. We are failing women postnatally, just as we are failing them in birth.

I asked a group of women via the Positive Birth Movement to describe their postnatal experience. There were many positives, but women also, somewhat reluctantly, admitted to 'putting on a front,' a kind of 'stiff upper lip' situation in which they rarely told others how they were really feeling. Some found that if they did tell others they were struggling this would immediately unleash a barrage of well-meant baby tips and advice, which they didn't want, as it only served to reinforce the idea that they 'weren't very good at this'. What they really wanted was practical support – someone to hold the baby while they showered or someone to make them a meal. Many described feeling lonely and isolated, in love with their baby but sometimes simultaneously bored of looking after them, which of course then led to feelings of guilt. Some, like Kate Scott-Clark from Exeter, felt that a traumatic birth compounded an already difficult situation: 'The loss of my old life coupled with this trauma felt like a bereavement. I just wanted the world to stop while I got to grips with all that had happened. I didn't want baby music, baby sensory or noisy toddler groups. I wanted someone else to say "fuck that was hard" and this is too.' Kate felt deskilled and hopeless at parenting, a sentiment echoed by another mum, Becca Bevis, who commented, 'My son's birth was full of interventions neither of us needed, which left me feeling utterly disempowered and doubting myself and my body. This definitely fed into how I was born as a mother, and the doubt in my instincts persisted for many months. I remember one midwife telling me crossly to "just smile – pretend if you have to" as tears poured on his cheeks from my eyes as I fed him. That felt like the proof I wasn't good enough and was getting it all wrong.'

# Seeing the water

Having a positive birth experience is not a solution to this postnatal crisis, but it might just help. We know that around 4 per cent of UK women each year report postnatal PTSD,[33] but the figures of women affected more mildly by birth trauma may be much higher. Still more may experience feelings of disempowerment, inadequacy, disappointment or sorrow that don't feel big or significant enough to report to a professional, but nevertheless affect women negatively as they begin the parenthood phase of their lives. And why? Because our current culture is geared towards this, it points women in this direction, carrying them along on a tide that they are repeatedly told is normal and then leaving them washed up on the deserted beach of new motherhood, shocked, battered, and lost. From the objectification of our bodies, to the media appetite for 'horror stories'; from the passive and soulless births on our TV screens, to the lack of positive attention given to new mothers; the maternity experience is, more often than not, a dehumanised one that we are persistently urged to be grateful for. As Marsden Wagner, Director of Women and Children's Health for the World Health Organisation, put it in the essay from which this chapter takes its name,[34] humanising birth is key: 'Humanising birth means understanding that the woman giving birth is a human being, not a machine and not just a container for making babies. Showing women – half of all people – that they are inferior and inadequate by taking away their power to give birth is a tragedy for all society. On the other hand, respecting the woman as an important and valuable human being and making certain that the woman's experience while giving birth is fulfilling and empowering is not just a nice extra, it is absolutely essential as it makes the woman strong and therefore makes society strong.'

The reason that birth is currently dehumanised, says Wagner, is because 'Fish can't see the water they swim in. Birth attendants, be they doctors, midwives or nurses, who have experienced only hospital-based, high-interventionist, medicalised birth cannot see the profound effect their interventions are having on the birth. These hospital birth attendants have no idea what a birth looks like without all the interventions, a birth which is not dehumanised.'

As women, and as feminists, we need to be the fish who see the water, and who keep describing it, loudly. We need to keep pointing out that birth can be different, that birth can be better, and that women care deeply about this life experience. We need to protest the sterile births on TV and demand that programme makers start to give more information about choice. We need to keep using social media to share alternative images and films of the kind of births that inspire us and make us proud. We need to share our stories, feelings and experiences in ways that feel uncensored, raw and brave. And we need to hold on to a vision of humanised birth, in which the woman is powerful and in control, and her physiology is trusted and respected. We know that not all birth can proceed without medical help, but even in those cases where intervention is truly needed, this can still be woman-centred and filled with humanity, as we will see in the next chapter which explores arguably the best hope we have of retaining a grip on humanised birth – by viewing it through the lens of human rights.

Chapter 7

# Birth Rights are Women's Rights are Human Rights

*I do not wish [women] to have power over men; but over themselves.*

Mary Wollstonecraft, *A Vindication for the Rights of Woman*[1]

In October 2013 I took a train from Somerset to London with a six-week-old baby strapped to my chest. Travelling with a tiny baby, I discovered, rather like having a puppy, is the ice-breaker that every socially anxious Brit is looking for, and literally everyone on my train greeted me with a warm, chatty curiosity that I've never experienced before or since on the UK transport system. They all wanted to know where I was going, and the answer was I was headed to give a short presentation at the 'Dignity in Childbirth' Forum, held by a new UK charity, Birthrights. Our conversations went something like this:

'Wow, on a train . . . he's so tiny! Where are you headed with such a small baby?'

'Um, I'm going to a conference, it's about human rights in childbirth.'

'Oh! Right! (pause) Human rights? In childbirth?'

'Yes!'

'So, like, what is that then? Is it about, like, people in, um, other countries?'

'No, not really! This event is all about the rights of UK women in the birth room.'

'Oh!'

Then would follow a stunned silence and more questions as each person I spoke to visibly tried to compute the concepts of 'human rights' and 'childbirth' – both of which they clearly had never heard placed side by side in a sentence before – and certainly not in the context of the UK maternity service. As the person trying to explain it to them (most often while a baby hoovered milk out of my boob in a busy train carriage), it was all relatively new to me, too. Although people had been talking about humanised birth, and reproductive rights for some time longer, the idea that a conversation needed to be had about the actual rights of women in the birth room itself was a fresh new thought.

So just what are a woman's rights in the birth room? The short answer is, as a global citizen, you have fundamental rights in childbirth just as you do in all other areas of your life. Applied to birth, your human rights include:

- the right to receive safe and appropriate maternity care
- the right to care that respects your dignity
- the right to privacy and confidentiality
- the freedom to make choices about your pregnancy and birth, even if your care providers don't agree with those choices
- the right to equality and freedom from discrimination

(source: Birthrights)[2]

# Free choices?

Much of this book has already been about human rights in childbirth, because feminism is about women's rights, and women are human. In the context of this book, the fourth point on the list above is perhaps particularly relevant: 'the freedom to make choices . . . even if your care providers don't agree'. Although it may sound fairly clear cut, in reality it appears to be a huge grey area of women's lives that is currently begging for feminist attention. As we have seen in countless examples throughout this book, women may be free to make their own choices in principle but, in reality, their freedom is highly dependent on several external factors such as geography, government funding, and – over and above anything else – the views of their care providers. These care providers may themselves be confused about the rights a woman has in the birth room and have a fear of litigation (rather than a woman's best interests) at the front of their minds, in particular if a woman wants to go 'against guidelines' or disagrees with their recommendations. One 2013 study published in the journal *BMC Pregnancy and Childbirth* found that professionals held conflicting beliefs about women's choices in childbirth;[3] on the one hand the health workers questioned stated that 'women were the ultimate decision makers', but also simultaneously agreed that 'the needs of the woman may be overridden for the safety of the fetus'. This was further complicated in the minds of the professionals by the belief that they themselves were ultimately legally accountable for outcomes of pregnancy and birth, despite the clear legal position that health care professionals are only liable for adverse outcomes caused by their own negligence.

The law is clear – women have bodily autonomy in pregnancy and birth just as they do at all other times in their lives, and they may not be compelled to undergo any procedure in birth – even if it would save their life or the life of their baby – any more than they may be compelled to have life-saving surgery or even to donate a kidney to save their dying twin. In parts of the world where there are 'grey areas' in the law around the right of the fetus to life or 'personhood' as it is sometimes called – which for obvious reasons are always interlinked with standpoints on termination of pregnancy, in turn often linked to strong religious views – we can see a direct and corresponding erosion of the rights of a woman to decide what happens to her own body. We've already heard the story of Adelir Carmen who was compelled to undergo a caesarean in Brazil in 2014 (see page 34). In the USA, at least 38 states have so-called 'fetal homicide' laws, which treat the fetus as separate from the woman who carries it, and therefore as a potential crime victim. The implications of this have included several hundred women in the USA being prosecuted and even jailed for pregnancy outcomes such as miscarriage or stillbirth. One woman, involved in a collision when drink-driving in New York that led to the death of two people in another car, was indicted on three counts of manslaughter – the two adults, and the unborn child she herself was carrying.[4] Another, from Iowa, spent two nights in jail after she fell down the stairs and confided to the emergency room nurse that she was struggling to cope in her pregnancy – a statement that the nurse interpreted as one of 'malicious intent'.[5] According to the *New York Times*, these and other similar cases 'illuminate a deep shift in American society, away from a centuries-long tradition in Western law and toward the embrace of a relatively new concept: that a fetus in the womb has the same rights as a fully formed person'.[6] Laws to protect the fetus are also used to regulate women's behaviour during pregnancy: women in at least 45 US states have faced criminal charges for drug use, while others face criminal regulation for drinking alcohol in pregnancy.[7]

If the state begins to regulate our pregnancy choices, where do we then draw the line? In the UK, the fetus does not have 'person-hood' and is not considered a person until birth, but could this ever change? In 2014, the English Court of Appeal ruled that a mother whose baby was born with fetal alcohol syndrome did not commit a crime,[8] in a case brought in an attempt to gain criminal injuries compensation. Significantly involved in the case were anti-abortion group the Pro-Life Research Unit, which former CEO of Birthrights, Rebecca Schiller, claims is a potential strategy to erode women's autonomy with the ultimate goal of criminalising termination: 'It's an almost inevitable attempt by the anti-abortion lobby to replicate their US colleagues' strategic claiming of pregnancy,' she says. Drinking alcohol in pregnancy may indeed be a 'bad choice', but supporting women to have the final say over what happens to their pregnant bodies is an 'all or nothing' situation in which, while we may not approve of 'bad choices,' we still have to support a woman's right to make them – that's how autonomy works.

Our nearest neighbours, Ireland, have only just repealed the Eighth Amendment, legislation that previously gave both mother and fetus equal rights – known for its impact on abortion but equally pervasive in the birth room. The Eighth may be repealed, but the attitudes that allowed the law to exist in the first place, themselves bound up in deeply held Christian values, continue across much of the island of Ireland, both north and south. When I marched for choice in Dublin in 2018, the placards summed up how women feel their physical autonomy has been eroded by Church and State: 'Keep Your Rosaries off My Ovaries,' 'Not Your Incubator,' 'Church and State Don't Ovulate,' 'Trust Women,' and, of course, 'My Body, My Choice'. An environment that does not fully trust women to make decisions about their own bodies will have a trickle-down effect into every interaction in maternity care. A midwife in a large hospital in Northern Ireland told me, 'Consent is incredibly important to me. I make sure and explain to women and their partners that they are the boss, and nothing happens to them without their say-so. Sadly, I seem to be virtually alone in that thinking. In my observation every day and every night women are having their human rights denied to them.'

Clearly there is confusion at a global level about women's rights in childbirth and their fundamental right to bodily autonomy, the legacy of a very long history of viewing women as objects, possessions, and reproductive vessels whose destiny and fate is up to men and God and upon which they are not to be consulted. While attitudes may slowly be changing, the confusion remains, and as a result, the imbalanced power dynamic of the birth room, in which women are given the general impression that they have agency but then find it is not actually there when they need it most, is perpetuated. As Hermine Hayes-Klein put it to me: 'How much would change in the birth room if everybody in that room really understood that the woman could not be touched without her permission – this would be transformative. And the fact that it would be transformative tells you everything you need to know about how informed consent is routinely ignored in current maternity care systems.'

## Birth rights in the zeitgeist

Hermine Hayes-Klein is an American lawyer who became interested in rights in birth when she had her own babies in the Netherlands, where she taught law at the Hague University and became Director of the Bynkershoek Institute's Research Center for Reproductive Rights. Although Hayes-Klein herself had positive home births with her midwife, Laura, she began to notice that even in the Netherlands, which has a reputation for a woman-centred attitude to birth, there were still increasing restrictions on women's freedom. Women were 'not allowed' to give birth at home with certain 'risk factors,' such as twin birth, and her own midwife, Laura, had faced charges for supporting women who wished to do so. 'When I gave birth to my babies, I thought I had a choice of where and with whom to give birth. But with these complaints against midwives for supporting other women's choices, I saw, Oh, I didn't choose, I was "allowed" while she's "not allowed",' Hermine told me. 'I realised that this is the bottom-line problem in the abuse of women during childbirth worldwide: confusion about whether women are capable adults making autonomous choices, or treated as incompetent or infantalised people whose informed reproductive choices are "allowed" or "not allowed".' As she researched the law around birth choices in the Netherlands, something extraordinary happened on the legal stage, the 2010 landmark case in the European Court of Human Rights (ECHR), known as Ternovskzy vs. Hungary.[9]

Pregnant with her second baby, Anna Ternovszky wanted a home birth, but knew her midwife, Agnes Gereb (see page 165), could face criminal charges, particularly in the case of a poor outcome, since the legal status of home birth in Hungary was ambiguous. Ternovszky accused the Hungarian state of violating two articles of the European Convention of Human Rights, one, Article 8, which asserts the right to privacy, and another which concerns anti-discrimination regulation. The ruling from the ECHR was that both of these rights had been violated. While the case was born out of a woman's desire to choose a home birth, the implications of the ruling are far wider, and affect every woman in her choices. The case was seen to establish in law a woman's right to choose how, where and with whom she gave birth – as the court ruling put it, 'The right concerning the decision to become a parent includes the right of choosing the circumstances of becoming a parent.' Ternovszky vs. Hungary is clear: the woman is the key decision maker in the birth room.

Something bigger and wider than the Ternovszky case was suddenly stirring into life. Inspired by the huge implications of the case for birth freedom, Hayes-Klein, in partnership with a group of Dutch birth activists known as Geboortebeweging,* convened the first Human Rights in Childbirth conference in The Hague, Netherlands in 2012. It was at this event that another lawyer, UK-based Elizabeth Prochaska, decided to found Birthrights, 'a place where the human rights principles and framework could be used to improve UK maternity care'. They launched in January 2013, just a few months after I myself had set up the Positive Birth Movement, although at the time we had never met and were not in touch. What we did have in common was more part of the zeitgeist – I hadn't been at the HRIC event in The Hague, but I had seen filmmakers Toni Harman and Alex Wakeford's *Freedom for Birth*,[10]

---

\*     Geboortebeweging, which translates as Birth Movement, was a group of around 50 birth activists who met for the first time in January 2011, out of concern for the increased medicalisation of childbirth. Hermine Hayes-Klein joined them at their third meeting. They are now a foundation promoting rights in birth in the Netherlands: http://geboortebeweging.nl

a documentary about the plight of Agnes Gereb, the Ternovszky case, and the wider restrictions all women face on their autonomy in the birth room which made a great impression on me. Harman and Wakeford organised over 1,000 screenings of their film in 50 countries and in 17 different languages on one day, 20 September 2012, and estimate that over 100,000 people saw the film that day – of which I was one. Wakeford said at the time of the film that he felt that medicalisation was to blame for the limits on freedom: 'Birth has been stolen, by a powerful institutionalised system that is born of fear, a system that inherently believes that birth is dangerous, and must be managed and controlled by modern technology.' Harman thinks that since they made the film, awareness of human rights in birth have improved 'significantly,' and remains hopeful that, with better staffing and resources, 'every expectant mother will be able to choose the circumstances of her birth, and those choices will be respected by every health professional.'

In many ways, Anna Ternovszky – who the majority of people will have never heard of – is an unsung hero. 'I am just like millions of other moms who wished to decide – and still hope to be able to do so in the future as well – where and under what conditions I would deliver my two babies,' she told the HRIC conference at The Hague, but in spite of this humility, she is not 'like millions of other moms' – for she is the one 'mom' who – along with Stefania Kapronczay and the Hungarian Civil Liberties Union – stood up and took direct and powerful action. This action has in turn been the catalyst for a whole chain of events that have transformed human rights in childbirth from a niche cause to a global movement. It's interesting to read the words Ternovszky used to describe her own birth experience, alongside those of HRIC's founder Hermine Hayes-Klein, which speak volumes about the impact of an empowering birth on women, and the confidence and motivating energy for change that such an experience can bring. There may not have been a ruling in the European Court or a major global conference on birth rights without Ternovsky or Hayes-Klein, but they may not have been motivated to take action without the strength they found in birth, and the deep bonds of loyalty they felt to their midwives:

> *I did not feel uncomfortable for a second, not even when I was on my hands and knees, yowling and writhing completely naked. I did not have to 'behave', nobody said anything – I felt accepted. I felt as if I was going to die from the pain, but feeling such faith from them (the midwives), knowing that they believed I could bear it, gave me tremendous strength, which was a very new feeling, something I enjoyed utterly. I had a chance to experience that I possess the ability to bring my child to this world by myself. I was given an opportunity to have a real meeting with myself and experience the immense power that lies within me. To this day it gives me great strength to recall and build upon that feeling.*
>
> Anna Ternovszky, 2012[11]

> *No matter how overwhelmed and out-of-control I felt, the faces surrounding me reflected peace and a quiet encouragement ... Nobody told me what to do, or*

*shouted 'push'. It would have been absurd; my body was doing the work, and I was only along for the ride. My body pushed, moved, and screamed when and how it needed to in order to give birth; any interference, orders, or restrictions would have obstructed the process and felt like torture ... Women talk about how childbirth can be a gate through which they pass into motherhood, and for me, this stage was that gate. My brain told me that what was happening was impossible, that the baby couldn't possibly fit out of me. I was afraid. As the baby came down, as he started to emerge, I looked to Laura (her midwife) and begged, 'Please! Get it out!' She looked me calmly in the eyes and said, 'I cannot do that for you. You need to push your baby out.' This was a life-changing moment for me. I realised, indeed, that only I could do this work, just as only I would mother this baby.*

Hermine Hayes-Klein, 2012[12]

With my third baby in my arms at the Birthrights conference, I had had two such birth experiences, at home, in a pool, with midwives who did nothing more than lock eyes with me in a gaze of deep trust when I needed them, and then stood well back while I got the job done myself. For me this also had a transformative power, changing the way I felt about myself, my body, my personal strength and my ability to face big challenges. It's perhaps easy, therefore, to see my move into the birth arena – and that of others like Hayes-Klein and Ternovszky – as simply a form of 'home birth evangelism'. Is this about every woman's right to the birth she wishes, or is it about a certain type of birth being held up as 'better' or 'best'?

## Birth rights for every birth

The wonderful thing about looking at birth through the lens of human rights is that it completely dispenses with these false dichotomies and demands instead that every woman is seen and supported as an individual. It is vital that we preserve and promote the widest possible range of options around place of birth and type of birth, for if the ability to make personal choices is diminished, we lose some of our collective freedom, even if the choices that were lost were not those we would have made ourselves. Knowing that we have the right to refuse treatment, for example, or that we can walk away and choose a different care provider, totally transforms the power dynamic in women's favour, even if they never choose to exercise that right. It's for this reason that we must unite as women and advocate for the right to every birth choice from unassisted home birth to elective caesarean – even if our own personal preference would be to have a hospital birth with an epidural, or to give birth via a surrogate, or not to have children at all. Part of 'giving birth like a feminist' lies in fighting for choices for our sisters and daughters that we wouldn't choose, wouldn't want, or might not even agree with ourselves.

# WHITE RIBBON ALLIANCE: RESPECTFUL MATERNITY CARE CHARTER.[13] THE UNIVERSAL RIGHTS OF CHILDBEARING WOMEN

In 2011, WRA launched a global campaign to promote a clear standard for respectful maternity care (RMC), rooted in international human rights. Working with global organisations, WRA produced the ground-breaking Respectful Maternity Care Charter, which has been translated into eight languages and continues to raise awareness and create policy change worldwide:

- Every woman has the right to be free from harm and ill treatment.
- Every woman has the right to information, informed consent and refusal, and respect for her choices and preferences, including the right to her choice

of companionship during maternity care, whenever possible.

- Every woman has the right to privacy and confidentiality.
- Every woman has the right to be treated with dignity and respect.
- Every woman has the right to equality, freedom from discrimination, and equitable care.
- Every woman has the right to healthcare and to the highest attainable level of health.
- Every woman has the right to liberty, autonomy, self-determination, and freedom from coercion.

If we think about birth in terms of the human right to choose, to be autonomous, and to experience humanised, personalised, and even 'loving' care, we can apply this to every single birth experience, shifting the focus away from 'mode of delivery' and towards how each individual woman is made to feel. This does not mean that we should lose sight of or stop celebrating women's natural birthing abilities, or refrain from discussing the effect of unnecessary intervention, however respectfully it is given. Respectful care for all does not negate the need to ensure that every woman who can have a straightforward birth, and wants one, gets one. Indeed, truly 'respectful' care surely means leaving behind any arrogant desire to control birth and giving a woman space and time to birth without unnecessary interference, just as true 'choice' means being able to choose unmedicated birth and being able to find a care provider who still has the confidence and skills truly to support that choice. For although much interesting and necessary dialogue can be found around a woman's right to choose caesarean, or epidural, or induction, we must not forget that in our current culture, a normal, straightforward, physiological birth is one of the hardest types of birth to come by, becomes rarer by the day, and is currently in danger of total extinction.

## Woman-centred obstetrics

What is also at risk of happening is women who, for whatever reason, can no longer have the straightforward birth they really wanted, feeling that they no longer have any rights or choices. As some put it, 'the birth plan went out the window'. On the contrary: when those situations that truly do require medical help arise, respectful care means continuing to keep women and their feelings at the heart of every action. Nothing illustrates this better than the many examples of clinicians trying to raise levels of empathy in highly medicalised settings. In Nottingham, obstetrician Andy Sim has been one of the pioneers of 'woman-centred caesarean,' which shifts the focus of surgical birth away from clinicians 'doing their job' and towards the woman as the pivotal character in the drama. This includes creating a peaceful atmosphere in the operating theatre with no 'chit chat,' playing music of choice, lowering the drapes so the woman and her partner can watch the birth, and facilitating delayed cord clamping and skin to skin. Of his work, Andy says, 'I think rather than seeing myself as someone who has made changes, I feel far more that I have changed to a position of much greater acceptance of women's choice.' One of Andy's 'small' changes – which of course any woman may ask to be part of her caesarean – is that, while the catheter is being inserted, theatre staff who are not needed for that procedure go and stand at the woman's head. When I've told people about this option, many will look a bit baffled and ask – why? Perhaps their first assumption is that there is a complex medical reason for the doctor's actions, but in fact the answer is simple – it's entirely about the woman's dignity. This seemingly small act of kindness says: 'We, the medical team, are thinking about what this is like for *you*, the person giving birth.' It's a sudden flash of empathy for how a woman, on the threshold of becoming a mother, may feel at that moment as an area of her body that is usually kept private is exposed. And it's an acknowledgement that in birth, everything is remembered, and everything 'matters'. Perhaps people are initially baffled by this because we're simply not used to the concept of building the activity in the birth room around the needs of the woman.

Thinking along similar lines, some NHS staff have taken the #lithotomychallenge, spending time on their back with their feet in stirrups in order to develop more empathy for the women in their care.[14] Obstetrician Florence Wilcock, who came up with the idea for the challenge as part of 'NHS Change Day' in 2015, spoke about how uncomfortable she found the experience, both physically and personally: 'My bottom (sacrum) was getting pretty sore and I had neck ache. My abdomen felt quite compressed and I thought if I was a woman in labour having to push it would probably make me feel quite nauseous . . . A midwife walked into the room with the door and curtain open and I realised I could see all the way down the corridor which meant everyone in the corridor could potentially see me . . . I was prepared to be filmed but it was interesting that a number of people walked in and out to look without talking to me . . . The camera man did a series of sound checks over me and proceeded to film without even speaking to me. I am sure it was an oversight but it gave me an amazing sense of being dehumanised.' Another team of health care professionals in Derby, known as 'Birth Outside the Box,' took the #theatrechallenge,[15] using film and role play to help clinicians experience being wheeled on a trolley to theatre, or the experience of caesarean. 'As the drapes went up, it made me feel that my body did not belong to me any more, I was powerless,' one participant commented. Other teams, such as St George's in Tooting, London, are developing ways to maintain a safe working environment while keeping the lights in theatre lower around the woman and her newborn – acknowledging the physical and psychological effects of dim lighting on oxytocin production, bonding, feeding, and the woman's personal experience and memory of the birth. And in Burnley, Lancashire, consultant obstetrician Liz Martindale has pioneered forceps and ventouse deliveries in which the woman, rather than being on her back, has been kneeling on the floor or in a standing position. 'In the first case of this kind, the woman had had a traumatic previous caesarean where she had felt she had no control or influence,' Liz told me. 'We were able to facilitate a birth using the "kiwi cup", with the patient leaning over the bed. She was delighted with her birth experience, particularly the fact that she was able to give birth in her chosen position and felt that she was empowered. Although safety of mother and baby are paramount, the effect of birth experience should always be considered,' Liz concludes.

## 'Gone are the days': the end of medical paternalism?

Central to any discussion about human rights in childbirth is the issue of consent. Another landmark case on maternity rights, known as Montgomery vs. Lanarkshire,[16] was heard in the UK Supreme Court in 2015, with great implications for consent, and described by one legal commentator as 'the belated obituary, not the death knell, of medical paternalism'.[17] The case concerned a woman – Mrs Montgomery – who was diabetic, meaning she had an increased risk of a shoulder dystocia in a vaginal birth. Her doctor felt that this risk was very small, and therefore decided not to inform Mrs Montgomery, feeling that if she told all diabetic women of this risk then, in her words, 'everyone would ask for a caesarean section'.

The court ruled that the doctor was wrong, and their ensuing guidance has much to tell us about birth as a feminist issue. Their ruling held that women have a right to information about 'any material risk' in order to make autonomous decisions about how to give birth. Supreme Court Justice Brenda Hale said, 'Gone are the days when it was thought that, on becoming pregnant, a woman lost, not only her capacity, but also her right to act as a genuinely autonomous human being.' The judgment called for dialogues about risk to be patient- or woman-centred – rather than asking themselves if their *medical colleagues* would feel a risk to be significant in a process known as the 'Bolam test,' doctors must ask if their *patient* would feel it to be significant. This demands more of doctors in terms of actually getting to know the pregnant woman in front of them as an individual, and trying to understand her more holistically. For example, the risks of complications for future pregnancies after a caesarean might be statistically small, but would be more *significant* to a woman who wanted to have a larger family than to a woman who didn't. Doctors must have conversations with their patients and these conversations must be a personalised, two-way dialogue, not just a delivery of a medical opinion or the passing on of a leaflet, said the ruling. Finally, and perhaps most importantly, a consent form alone is not enough: 'The doctor's duty is not therefore fulfilled by bombarding the patient with technical information which she cannot reasonably be expected to grasp, let alone by routinely demanding her signature on a consent form.'

The Montgomery ruling is powerful stuff. It has demanded a shake-up of medical thinking that is still, at the time of writing, taking time to settle. For some, it has raised concerns about the level of information given to women and where to 'draw the line,' while others worry that the ruling will increase litigation – both such concerns exposing the lack of consideration for women's intelligent autonomy upon which so much of maternity care has been built. Women are, as they always have been, keen to be treated as adults and given personalised, clear information upon which to make their decisions – decisions for which, given this proper information, they are happy to take personal responsibility. A group of experts convened by Birthrights as part of the Sheila Kitzinger Programme at Green Templeton College Oxford,[18] explored the issues raised by the ruling, concluding that, going forwards, 'There was a need to articulate why informed consent was important – it is not only a legal requirement, and an ethical imperative to uphold the rights of birthing women as equal citizens, but it is what women want, and results in safer, personalised and less traumatic care.' They also recognised that, 'paternalism still existed and [that there was] work to be done before informed consent was universally understood and practised.' The group considered how health professionals could be helped to retain their humanity and ability to understand a woman's perspective, and wondered, 'How could we banish the language of allowed/not allowed?' Clearly the Montgomery ruling is demanding important questions be asked about rights-based, woman-centred care.

Montgomery also quite rightly demands that women are given as much information as possible and are placed at the centre of decision making. Across the world, the principle of medical consent has always been built upon a clinician giving information. We cannot legally consent to something happening to our bodies without being given the proper information – in other words, if it is not 'informed consent' it is not consent at all. In relation to childbirth, some raise the issue of 'capacity' – this means that a health professional can make decisions for you if it is felt that you do not have the 'capacity' to make those decisions yourself. The idea that a woman in the throes of labour might not be able to make decisions for herself is suggested more frequently than you would hope, and this is probably connected to the idea that pregnancy and motherhood themselves diminish a woman's capability to think and be rational (as indeed does simply being female: the word 'hysterical' comes from the Greek for womb and literally means your uterus is causing you to behave illogically). I'll never forget the moment, in my first pregnancy, that I was accused in a very serious work meeting of having 'baby brain,' a condition which doesn't have much scientific backing, but which is used to discredit women's opinions nevertheless. To question the 'capacity' of a woman in labour shows both a misunderstanding of the concept of capacity itself and of what being in labour is actually like. Struggling, feeling exhausted, upset, in pain, overwhelmed or desperate for the whole thing to be over may indeed be how you are feeling in the final hours before you meet your baby, but they do not mean that your mind is not functioning to the extent that you are unable to make decisions. In order to lack capacity in the law, you would normally have to be heavily intoxicated with drugs or alcohol, brain damaged by a stroke or other injury, be severely learning disabled, suffer from dementia, have a condition that was causing confusion or a loss of consciousness, or suffer from a severe mental health condition such as schizophrenia.[19] If none of these applied to you before you went into labour, it is very unlikely that the experience of being in labour itself will cause you to lose capacity. Nor is it automatically the case that you 'lack capacity' if you wish to make a decision about your care that others do not agree with. If it is felt that you are truly unable to make decisions, then your partner and, if possible, your birth plan should be consulted, and any intervention must be in your best interests.

> *You have the right to accept or refuse treatment that is offered to you, and not to be given any physical examination or treatment unless you have given valid consent. If you do not have the capacity to do so, consent must be obtained from a person legally able to act on your behalf, or the treatment must be in your best interests.*
>
> From the NHS Constitution[20]

# 'It needed to be finished'

While being in labour itself does not usually mean that your mind is not functioning properly, what many women do report is that they no longer wish to have conversations or dialogue with any other person, and that they find it deeply distracting. Women often speak of labour as a kind of 'other worldly' place, 'labourland,' a kind of meditative or trance-like state. Being asked questions is particularly unpleasant in that it 'breaks the spell' and draws you back into the modern, analytical neocortex part of your brain when you very much need to be using your mammalian, limbic area. So although you usually have 'capacity' in labour, I do think you become more vulnerable to being *coerced* into decisions that don't actually feel right to you, for the simple reason that you do not wish to enter into prolonged debate or respond to persistent questioning. There is therefore a need for the conversation around consent in childbirth to shift focus away from a woman's possible inability to make decisions, and on to the way health professionals interact with that woman, what information they impart, when they impart it, and – perhaps most importantly – their own ability to accept a woman's right to decline. Too many birth stories are currently filled with women who felt they had to 'give in' to pressure placed on them to make certain decisions that they did not want but that professionals clearly felt were in their best interests. Too many women report their choices not being framed as choices at all, but rather as 'assertions': 'We need you to get on the bed now,' 'I'm just going to examine you' and so on. Lack of consent is not always black and white – sometimes it's a clear and horrifying violation, but other times it comes in the form of a 'brisk bedside manner' that is harder to identify in the moment. You may be told that you 'need to' get on the bed, or that something is 'going to' happen next, and only afterwards have time to reflect that you did not really get given the option to decline. You may only find out after the birth that something happened against your wishes, for example your baby's cord being cut while you yourself were distracted or receiving other treatment, or having been given an episiotomy. You may feel coerced, for example by being told that your baby 'may die' but not being given any more information or time to ask more questions. Women frequently report their partners being drawn in to the coercion: 'Convince your wife to listen,' one woman in Croatia said her partner was told. Georgie Watson gave birth in Cornwall in 2013, and says she was made to get out of the pool for a vaginal exam. 'I didn't want the exam, but she told my husband she couldn't tell if the baby was breech and that "would be extremely dangerous". My husband panicked and asked me to get out of the pool, even though he knew I didn't want to and he knew my baby wasn't breech. I was then subjected to a brutal VE fully dilated, while contracting and my waters were forcibly broken. It ruined my birth and psychologically affected me and my husband for a long time.'

Of note is that Georgie did try to complain about her experience, but the midwife she raised her concerns with defended the birth midwife's actions. 'No VE is pleasant, if she had stopped when you had asked I doubt you would have let her continue the examination, and it needed to be finished,' Georgie was told.

The professional emphasis here, as it is so often, is on what they needed to do in order to 'do their job' rather than any consideration for the woman's experience. Georgie and her needs are completely invisible in the midwife's words. 'I began to doubt myself, as if maybe I had remembered wrong or was overreacting,' she told me. 'But I have gone on to become chair of my local Maternity Voices Partnership, determined to change this.' Stories like hers, in which a clear understanding of consent is entirely absent, make difficult reading, but are important to air, not least because the notion that the violation of women's rights in childbirth is something that happens 'elsewhere' and not in the privileged 'developed' world, is all too prevalent. Perhaps, too, we should not be entirely surprised that this disregard for women's bodily autonomy takes place, when there is still huge work to be done on the wider issue of consent. A 2018 survey by the End Violence Against Women Coalition and YouGov found that many people's understanding of what constitutes rape is very unclear: a third of men in Britain believe that if a woman has flirted on a date it 'generally wouldn't count as rape' even if she didn't explicitly consent to sex, and 33 per cent believe it 'isn't usually rape' if a woman is pressured into sex without 'physical violence' taking place.[21] Birth and sex are both intimate physical experiences in which a loss of control, trust and agency feel deeply violating, yet in both there seems to be a flagrant disregard for a woman's body boundaries, and a massive cultural deaf-spot when a woman quite clearly says, 'No.'

At the Birthrights Dignity in Childbirth Forum I attended with my newborn baby, they unveiled the results of their 2013

Dignity Survey,[22] undertaken in partnership with the parenting website Mumsnet. Overall, 12 per cent of respondents felt that they had not given their consent to examinations and procedures, with the number being higher again in first-time mothers (16 per cent), and higher still (23 per cent) for those who gave birth in hospital (as opposed to a midwife-led unit). Highest of all was the number of women who had had an instrumental birth – 24 per cent of them said that their consent had not been obtained. Similar figures were produced by a 2016 survey from Positive Birth Movement and Channel Mum: over 22 per cent of the 2,186 women who responded did not feel that they consented to everything but were instead told that they 'had to' have certain procedures.[23] And in the USA, a 2013 survey by Childbirth Connection found that 6 out of 10 episiotomies were performed without consent.[24] Cristen Pascucci, who is making a film about consent in US childbirth called 'Mother May I?,'[25] says, 'Consent is a key issue in this human rights crisis. When I was pregnant, many of the messages I received were intended to encourage a compliant patient, not an informed and active participant. My mission is to flip the system upside down so that women and birthing people are on top.'

# MAKING A COMPLAINT ABOUT YOUR CARE

If women don't give feedback about their birth experience, nothing will change. Positive feedback is vital. If you feel you had fantastic care, from care providers who truly listened to you, treated you as an individual and with respect and dignity, then it's helpful to let them know so that they can see just how much this made a difference to you and your family. By the same token, it's really important to raise your voice if you feel you could have had a better birth. This might be just general reflections on what could have been improved, or specific complaints about incidents in which you felt there was an unnecessary lack of choice, disrespectful treatment or a violation of your body boundaries. You may even want to report an individual practitioner to their professional body, or take legal action. Whatever the nature of your complaint, raise your voice. You can't change what happened to you, but you might change birth for women of the future.

- You have the right to make a formal complaint about your care. For regional organisations who can give you more advice and support in your actions see the

Resources section at the back of this book.

- If you wish to complain about your maternity care before you give birth, speak to your midwife or doctor or their manager or supervisor. If you don't feel you are getting the response you hope for, take your complaint higher – to regional or national managers.
- If your complaint concerns your birth experience, try to jot down everything you can remember about it as soon as you possibly can. You may forget some details and they will be very useful in any complaints procedure. If you find this process upsetting, take your time and seek support.
- Ask anyone who attended the birth with you to make a note of some key points about what they remember, too.
- Try to obtain a copy of your maternity notes as soon as you possibly can. In most parts of the world, you have a legal entitlement to obtain them. Once you have had time to look over the copy of your notes, you may also wish to attend the hospital to view the originals and check that nothing has been omitted from the copy.
- You may wish to make an informal complaint to your hospital or care providers, or you may wish to make a formal complaint. To find out where to send a formal letter of complaint, ask your health care provider. This may be the chief executive of the hospital or other

senior figures. You may also like to complain to an individual's professional body. You may wish to copy in your Member of Parliament, the ombudsman or national body who represents patients in your area, and any other professionals or organisations who you feel should know about your situation.

- When writing your letter of complaint, numbered bullet points are helpful and will enable you to be clear, when you get a response, which points (if any) they have not addressed.

- If you are invited to a meeting to discuss your complaint, take someone with you. Take notes of every response to your complaint and of what is said at any meeting, and keep these safe.

- There may be a time limit within which you can make your complaint, for example within 12 months of the birth. If you wish to complain outside of this time limit, do so anyway. It is still important to make your voice heard and give your feedback.

- If you feel there may be cause for legal action against your care provider, seek legal advice.

- If you complain through all the appropriate channels and still feel that your complaint is not being heard, you may wish to speak using social media. This can be an effective way of finding others who have been in a similar position to you, and of raising awareness of poor treatment.

# Having a voice is a privilege

While the data we have around consent is already worrying, I feel that the actual numbers may be even higher, since women who respond – for example, to a survey about 'dignity in childbirth' – may already have a fairly good sense of their rights. As we have seen elsewhere in this book, it is the 'middle-class birthzillas' who often receive the worst criticism for their 'laminated birth plans' – but perhaps they are just tricky customers because they know more about what they are entitled to. If you are reading this book, you may even be one of them. More marginalised women, with less access to education, information and support, may not only not be picking up this book in Waterstones or responding to an online Mumsnet survey, but may also not realise that they did not consent to procedures in childbirth because they did not know that they had a choice in the first place. Doulas – wrongly considered by some to be another preserve of the privileged – often work voluntarily with marginalised groups, supporting them and protecting their rights. Maddie McMahon works as a volunteer doula with the Cambridge Refugee Resettlement Campaign, and agrees that there can be even greater barriers than usual to respectful care: 'Most of the time, the most an asylum seeker can expect from the NHS is a translator on the end of the phone. It's not a 24/7 service and you often have to wait. A combination of language barriers, lack of antenatal education and often no continuity of carer, means they often have very little choice or ability to advocate for themselves. But what annoys me the most is the apparent inability to take into account that these women have probably been traumatised, and medical interventions may well trigger them deeply.' Katie Olliffe, from Cambridge, works for Birth as a Medium for Change, who provide vulnerable and socio-economically disadvantaged women in the local community with doulas. 'I find that they are inclined to believe they have no choice,' she told me. 'They are already vulnerable and disempowered either from having social services involvement or the (perceived) threat of social services involvement, and already feeling as though they have to do as they are told and feeling judged for their complex issues, for example mental health, domestic violence or addiction.' Doulas who work with vulnerable women play a vital role in supporting their human rights, empowering them to ask questions and challenge things they are uncomfortable with, and helping them to have the voice that many of us take for granted.

Birth Companions[26] is a charity that works to improve the lives of pregnant women and new mothers facing severe disadvantage. Their volunteers and staff offer practical and emotional support, including birth support, to women in prison and the community. I asked their director, Naomi Delap, for her view on the human rights in childbirth of the women they work with. 'At Birth Companions we see frequent examples of the challenges that compromise the intrapartum care of women facing severe disadvantage, including perinatal women in prison,' she told me. 'These include not giving women adequate information and support in order to give informed consent to procedures and not protecting women's privacy and confidentiality. There is also a lack of understanding of the impact of women's past experiences and circumstances on their experiences of care and their outcomes, particularly around lifetime and birth trauma. Shockingly, women experiencing multiple challenges – those in most need – are shown through the evidence base to have the worst experiences of care and the poorest outcomes. This is something that urgently needs to be addressed at every level within maternal health and the wider systems within which women are cared for.'

We know that black women in the USA are three to four times more likely[27] to die in pregnancy and birth than their white counterparts, and the latest figures from MBRRACE show that in the UK, their mortality rate is five times higher.[28] Candice Brathwaite, founder of Make Motherhood Diverse, feels that black women are simply not listened to in their maternity care, due to a racial bias that is often subconscious. 'After the birth of my own daughter, I knew there was something wrong – my c-section wound was swollen and I kept sweating right through to the mattress – but I felt my concerns were not listened to. This was not a new experience, as I had felt very similarly during birth, when I was treated as if the pain was "only in my head". When I was finally rushed to hospital with acute sepsis, I actually felt like I had won. I now had evidence that something wasn't right. Upon reflection, I see how lucky I am. There are many more black women who die because when they speak about how they feel, they aren't believed – and it's so great that we now have the data to support what we already knew.' A 2013 survey of US maternity care, 'Listening to Mothers III,' revealed that one in five black and Hispanic women reported poor treatment from hospital staff due to race, ethnicity, cultural background or language, as compared to one in twelve white women.[29] If black women are not being listened to in their births, you can be sure that their human rights are not being respected, their consent is not being properly sought, and their birth preferences are being ignored. Just like white women then – except with an added layer of racism, and therefore at even higher proportions.

It's beyond the scope of this book to give a comprehensive world picture of birth, but nevertheless, as feminists, we might like to consider a few more global examples of care that flagrantly disregard human rights. Natalia de Biegler runs a Positive Birth Movement group in Guatemala City, and told me, 'Most women give birth in public or private hospitals, with doctors. Almost all birthing women have to lie down to push because of hospital policies. The 'Kristeller manoeuvrer'* is still routine practice here. It is sad and very frustrating to see women being coerced into making decisions they don't want to, out of fear and guilt. There is lack of respect, little space for choice, and a lot of obstetric abuse going on. In fact, it was because of these issues that I decided to become a doula and advocate for birth rights, but let me tell you, it has been uphill. It's heartbreaking.' A similar report comes from Sara Vale who runs Positive Birth Movement Lisbon: 'Obstetric violence is still rampant in Portuguese hospitals, and real evidenced-based information does not reach the vast majority of women. Also, a deeply ingrained cultural belief that "doctor knows best" is still predominant in Portuguese

---

* Pressure is applied to the fundus (bump) during the 'pushing stage'– many experts have serious concerns about the safety of this practice to mother and baby.

society. Most women don't know they can refuse procedures. They just accept it. Maternity services do not encourage shared decision making and inquisitive women. And that is what is so perverse: obstetric violence is so ingrained that women expect it and endure it.' And in India, the Facilitator of Positive Birth Movement Chennai, Sangeetha Parthasarathy, tells me, 'Essentially you are talking about a misogynistic, patriarchal culture where women are treated as vessels to produce (preferably male) offspring. Even urban educated women would actually do a double take when you tell them they have choices in maternity. The typical birth is a C-section – around 80 per cent of babies are born this way in urban India. Or an over-medicalised horrendously traumatic vaginal birth which women call "Normal Delivery" – Routine IV fluids on admission, enema, shaving between legs, lithotomy, CTG, Pitocin, vaginal exams every half or one hour, routine episiotomy especially for first-time mothers, fundal pressure during pushing (especially in state-funded hospitals), and then rushing for an emergency C-section. There is some activism following the Human Rights in Childbirth conference being held in Mumbai in 2017, but I can tell you we are all exhausted from the sheer magnitude of what's going on.'

## Sing loud like canaries

Women who face these terrifyingly limited choices will sometimes choose to birth alone rather than risk giving birth in hospital. This is why Brigid McConville of the White Ribbon Alliance says, 'Respectful maternity care in hospital settings is vital to safe motherhood, because if women are afraid to go to hospital to give birth, they will do so outside of hospital. Unless they live in a place which provides skilled midwifery care at home, that has its own set of risks.' Around the world, however, in every country, more and more women, even those with the option of home birth midwives, are making the choice to avoid formal medical care for their births entirely. Professor of Midwifery Hannah Dahlen calls these women 'the canary in the coal mine'. 'Women's rights to choice, respect and evidence-based care are not being met in many countries around the world,' Dahlen, who is writing a book about her research with women choosing to birth outside the system, told me. 'Women are increasingly voting with their feet and choosing to give birth outside mainstream care in order to avoid systems that have traumatised them during previous births or during current maternity care interactions. It is time we wake up as maternity health care providers and take a long hard look at what we are doing to women in childbirth and the limited options we are providing them with. These women are not "mad" and they are not "bad" as is so often alleged. After interviewing and surveying thousands of women who choose to birth outside the system it is clear they love their babies as much as women who give birth in the system but they see birth in the system as unsafe, both physically and psychologically for themselves and their babies. If we don't listen to these women and hear what they are trying to tell us it will be to everyone's detriment.'

Human rights is not a competition. As the saying goes, 'Equal rights for others does not mean less rights for you – it's not pie.'

Likewise, having more rights than others doesn't mean you should be content simply on the basis that someone else is worse off. Western women who complain about their maternity care are often paternalistically reminded to 'remember how lucky they are,' in comparison to the atrocious birth experiences of women elsewhere in the world, or of a different socio-economic status, or of a different ethnicity. This has a silencing effect, rather like telling the woman who has been assaulted on the bus home, 'You're lucky you didn't get raped.' No, she is not lucky. Nobody who is hurt or violated in any way, however great or small, is 'lucky,' nor should they be silent about it. Regardless of where on the spectrum of disrespectful maternity care we find ourselves, the fact that 'other women have it worse' does not mean we should keep quiet about our own situation. As women I think we are taught from a young age to diminish our discomfort. Even our shoes and our clothing are impractical and uncomfortable, and the majority of men would not tolerate wearing them for five minutes. If we are sexually harassed, or even assaulted, we may tell ourselves, 'It's not that serious, worse things happen to other women, probably nobody will believe me, maybe I'm exaggerating it in my mind' and so on. What #metoo has shown us is not only the enormous numbers of women who have been diminishing their discomfort and keeping quiet about it, but also the power of the collective voice, and that every story, however 'small,' is worth telling. There is a snowball effect of so many stories all slowly sticking to each other and gathering in one place, and a feeling of 'safety in numbers' for the tellers. We must not ignore what is happening to all women in childbirth, regardless of how small or 'not worth mentioning' we feel the incidents of disrespect to be. Speaking out raises the issue for us, for other women in our own country, and helps in the global struggle for all women, everywhere, to be treated with dignity and autonomy in childbirth.

Since I caught that train with my newborn boy, the landscape of human rights in childbirth has been rapidly changing. There have been some retrograde steps – two other cases[30] in the European Court, for example, have found that the denial of the choice of home birth does not violate Article 8's right to privacy, in contrast with the landmark ruling of Ternovszky. Another case, however, has found that a woman who had medical students present at her birth against her wishes did have her human right to privacy violated.[31] It feels like even the European Court of Human Rights themselves are still finding women's choice a complex area to navigate. In the USA, two landmark cases, that of Kimberly Turbin (see page 46) and Caroline Malatesta, who won a $16-million law suit for her mistreatment in childbirth,[32] have unleashed another flood of women's stories and an energetic movement towards change. Many organisations are working globally with human rights in childbirth high on their agenda, from grassroots movements, to region-specific initiatives (see Resources), to the World Health Organisation, who have said that, 'Respectful maternity care – which refers to care organised for and provided to all women in a manner that maintains their dignity, privacy and confidentiality, ensures freedom from harm and mistreatment, and enables informed choice and continuous support during labour and childbirth – is recommended.'[33] The White Ribbon Alliance is running a 2019 campaign called What

Women Want,[34] which Brigid McConville, Creative Director of WRA UK, says will ask a million women about their own maternity priorities: 'It's astounding how many of those women have expressed surprise at even being asked, as if it's a given they have no say in what happens to their own bodies during pregnancy and birth. Which of course is all too often the reality. By challenging that we are challenging the power structures that still subjugate women by denying their reproductive rights, choices, autonomy – all around the world.' As more and more women open up about 'what they want,' and how their birth experiences made them feel, using hashtags like #exposingthesilence, #breakingthesilence, #metoo and #metoointhebirthroom, the collective voice is growing louder. I now wish I could go back and explain to the people who asked me on that train just what exactly human rights in childbirth meant. If I had time, I'd tell them everything I've told you in this chapter, but if their stop was approaching and I had to be brief, I would simply say, 'Women have the human right to be the key decision maker over what happens to their body, and to be listened to, and treated with respect. They've been denied that right for a while now, so they've decided to rise up and claim it. It's that simple.'

# Chapter 8

# What Women Want. What Women Need. What Women Are.

*One of the most deplorable cases in all the present calamity was that of women with child, who, when they came to the hour of their sorrows, and their pains come upon them, could neither have help of one kind or another; neither midwife or neighbouring women to come near them.*

A Journal of the Plague Year (1722), Daniel Defoe[1]

Much has happened in the three years since the first edition of *Give Birth Like a Feminist* was published. First and foremost, a global pandemic, an unprecedented event that seemed to knock everything we held familiar or took for granted completely off its axis. Secondly, while my own world shrank down to teaching three children maths at the kitchen table, I simultaneously branched out and wrote a book for preteen girls about periods, which enabled me to offer a new and more positive narrative to young girls about their female bodies. During this time there was a third event of note – a distinct increase in temperature in the so-called 'gender wars', and a volatile debate about what it means to be a woman, which in 2020 caught me directly in its crossfire.

There is a thread that runs through all three – pandemic, periods and the debates around gender: a sidelining of women and their needs, a kind of collective dismissal of our importance as fully formed, whole humans. This is the same dismissal you have read about again and again in the pages of this book; it is woven through women's history, and through the experience of childbirth itself.

# What is essential?

The pandemic has had an impact on every area of our lives, including, of course, health care. In the UK and elsewhere, health services were forced to stretch even further to accommodate rising numbers of Covid cases, and to incorporate new infection-control procedures. Frontline running costs in the NHS have been estimated to have increased by £4–5 billion a year,[2] and waiting lists for treatment swelled from 4.3 million in January 2020, to nearly 6.5 million in April 2022.[3]

This impact included, of course, maternity care. The immediate message pregnant women were given was that maternity services had to be 'pared back to the essentials'. At first glance, in particular against the wider backdrop of suffering brought on by Covid, this may seem sensible and fair, but a deeper exploration reveals that what made the list of 'essentials' says a lot about how the maternity system views what is essential or not when it comes to women and their needs. Health care providers worked under unimaginably difficult circumstances and it's important to be clear that it's the wider maternity system and culture that I'm critiquing here, rather than individuals within it. And when we look at this wider system, it can't be denied that the parts that were pared back were often those which provide women with reassurance and comfort, increase their autonomy and choice, and raise their chance of a positive experience of birth. These, apparently, were not 'essential'.

Home birth, birth in a midwife-led unit and water birth were, of course, the first to be stopped or restricted, as was maternal-request caesarean. Often with no alternative but to birth in hospital, women then faced restrictions over who would be allowed to accompany them during labour or on the postnatal ward, with some trusts saying that women could not have a partner with them at all, in particular if they tested positive. Many women had to attend scans alone, and in situations where, for example, they were given difficult news about their baby's wellbeing, they felt incredibly isolated. Face-to-face antenatal and postnatal appointments with midwives and other health professionals were ended for the majority of women. In September 2020, you could visit a pub with five friends but your partner could not attend a scan with you. You could have a wedding with up to 30 guests, but only one birth partner was allowed at the birth of your baby (it was common for women to be told that they could only have one person with them during labour, which in real terms meant that doulas were not considered essential, and that, given that the majority of women would choose to have their partner with them, neither were mothers, best friends, sisters or any other support people).

Although in the UK pandemic restrictions were lifted in February 2022, during the following month of March, many of these restrictions remained in place, with women in some parts of the UK still having to attend scans alone, and having limited access to their partner or other birth support during labour, and postnatally – in spite of the fact that almost all other pandemic restrictions had been lifted. At the time of writing, some restrictions still remain and continue to fluctuate, with some areas stopping and then reintroducing mask use, for example, with other restrictions continuing on visitors and options like home birth.

Throughout the pandemic, campaign group #ButNotMaternity have called for maternity care to be treated differently to other medical care, emphasising that birth is more of a celebratory life event than a medical procedure, and pointing out unfairness and discrepancy.[4] To date, nearly 700,000 people have signed a petition asking for all Covid-related maternity restrictions to be lifted.[5]

Covid safety was also used to further justify routine vaginal exams, an area of maternity care that even pre-pandemic was fraught with issues around women's bodily autonomy and consent. In the 2019 edition of this book, I had discussed the issues around routine checks on cervical dilation (see pages 37–39), and how pregnant women were often made to feel that VEs were compulsory, when of course they are not (and nobody should ever be made to feel like this is the case when it comes to an internal exam). Even in a pre-Covid world, some women were being 'persuaded' by being told, 'We need to know how dilated you are before you can be admitted,' or 'You need a vaginal exam before you get in the pool.' This coercion, which often involved gatekeeping something a woman desperately wanted or needed in exchange for her compliance, went up a gear in the pandemic and it soon became, 'You can't have your partner by your side until you are 4cm.'

The group Pregnant Then Screwed surveyed over 15,000 women who gave birth between March and November 2020 and found that one in five of them felt they had no choice but to have a vaginal exam, with four out of five women agreeing to exams in order to then be allowed to have their partner join them.[6] At the time, I spoke to some women who had personally experienced this. Ruth, who gave birth in London, told me, 'I tried to refuse the VE but the hospital threatened to send my partner home. In the end I gave in and let them but it felt very violating.' Anna said, 'I went to the hospital in the middle of the night twice. I was in early labour, contracting, and my partner had to wait at the door. Both times I was examined, alone, found not to be dilated enough and sent home. It felt pretty horrendous and inhumane.' And Ali: 'I was told my partner had to stay outside until they had 'diagnosed' labour. It was absolutely not presented as something I had any say in whatsoever. If I wanted my partner, I had to go through it.'[7]

Their stories seem shocking, but even before the pandemic, there were serious issues around VEs and consent. A 2016 survey from Positive Birth Movement and Channel Mum found that over a third of women didn't know that they had the right to decline vaginal exams, with over 20 per cent reporting that they were told they 'had to' have certain procedures and that their consent was not sought.[8] Withholding a woman's partner from her in labour unless she consents is a particularly barbaric form of coercion, but it was arguably only made possible by attitudes deeply embedded in maternity care long before any of us had ever heard of the coronavirus. When I was asked to discuss these enforced VEs on BBC Radio 2's Jeremy Vine show in November 2020, one (male) caller said, 'Giving birth is not a time to worry about being examined.' Yet again the majority view seems to be that any usual expectations about bodily autonomy or consent become ridiculous once you are in labour, because 'all that matters is a healthy baby'. In reality, putting fingers into a woman using coercion in this way is illegal and could constitute battery, but a lawsuit seems unlikely while most people continue to believe that such treatment is perfectly justifiable.

Some women during the pandemic have chosen to 'vote with their feet', and birth at home. According to the Office for National Statistics, in the UK the numbers of women giving birth at home during the first year of Covid rose by 7 per cent, from 13,407 homebirths in 2019 to 14,281 in 2020.[9] And in the USA, the numbers of home births rose by nearly 20 per cent, from 38,000 in 2019 to 45,000 in 2020, according to the US Centers for Disease Control and Prevention.[10] Several UK mothers in a home birth group told me they only got their home birth through sheer willpower: 'I point blank refused to go into hospital and they eventually sent a midwife' was the recurring theme.

It would be interesting to know the numbers of women who would have chosen to home birth had all the services remained available. The extra restrictions in place for birth partners, coupled with other concerns about leaving home during lockdown and exposing themselves, their family or their baby to Covid, meant that home birth appealed to those who might not have previously considered it. However, for many, it was simply not an option. In early 2020, NHS trusts in the UK began to suspend home birth services, citing a shortage of midwives and maternity support workers. According to a March 2020 survey from the RCM, 32 per cent of heads of midwifery reported a stop to their home birth service. This trend continued throughout the pandemic – in November 2021, for example, an investigation by the *Observer* found that more than twenty trusts across the UK had had disrupted home birth services in the previous three months, with eight confirming their services remained fully suspended due to staff shortages.[11]

For those who had the funds, private midwifery services were appealing. In 2019 the UK company Private Midwives had 209 women book a home birth; in 2020 that figure more than doubled to 423. Private Midwives also offer a service of antenatal and postnatal appointments only, with no attendance at the birth itself, which 87 women booked in 2019. In 2020 that number doubled, and in 2022 it tripled.[12] Women wanted time and full attention from their care providers, and were prepared to pay for it. 'The key factors that are important to women are time, and choice,' Linda Bryceland, their director, told me. 'Women are fed up with antenatal appointments that they have to take half a day off work for but that only last ten minutes with someone who doesn't have time to listen to them. They also often feel like their choices are not respected by the NHS. The partner restrictions on top of this have also been a huge issue.'

Some without access to a private midwife have turned to freebirth, with one in twenty expectant women considering birthing without a doctor or midwife present, according to one study conducted in July 2020[13] – up 3 per cent on 2019. Beverley Turner had an unassisted birth at home in Stoke-on-Trent in September 2021, at which point home births in her area were suspended. 'My partner was present from start to finish with our first child's labour', she told me. 'My opinion is that the child I bear is as much the father's as it is mine, and I don't think their involvement should be dictated to them by medical professionals. I also didn't understand the Covid policies, which said that my partner could come and "settle me in" and then would have to go away and come back later when I was in "established labour". Surely it would be more dangerous for somebody to leave the premises and then come back because in that time they could have come into contact with somebody with Covid?'

Louise Day, who had a freebirth in Scotland in 2020, felt similarly about the Covid risks. 'I felt more at risk of catching the virus in the hospital as I'd come into contact with more staff,' but she was also motivated by difficult experiences in her previous birth: 'I didn't feel I consented to some things in my first birth in hospital and I didn't want to face that again.' Consent was an issue of key concern for both women. Beverley said, 'I didn't want VEs through my labour anyway, so there was no way I was having a VE just to determine if I could have my partner by my side – which is also why I decided to stay at home.' Louise agreed: 'In my first birth, I was told, "Just hop up on the bed and we'll examine you" and ended up having a VE I didn't want or need. When I heard I would have to have one in this labour just to have my partner with me, I decided I didn't want to have that argument or discussion.'

## What is needed?

Whether from Covid or from violating examinations, labouring women need to feel safe, and this is a deep, mammalian need. We know that women cannot give birth vaginally without the hormone oxytocin. We know that this is the 'shy hormone', and that it needs darkness, privacy and a warm, loving environment to flourish. And we know that the 'fight or flight' hormone adrenaline, produced when we feel threatened or afraid, can inhibit the production of oxytocin. In Chapter 4, we looked at how labouring women have basic needs, and to put it simply, the most ideal birth environment is one in which we'd like to have romantic sex. 'The same energy that gets the baby in, gets the baby out', as the saying goes.

It only took me a paragraph to explain that to you, but these absolute basics of female physiology have been ignored for decades now, with birth rooms built with the needs of care providers in mind, rather than the needs of women. Bright lights so the birth attendants can see, beds so the birth attendants can reach, open doors so the birth attendants can come and go as they please – all of these standard elements of birth room architecture centre the care provider over the production of oxytocin, in spite of the mechanics of this hormone being so obvious and so basic.

The pandemic has no doubt exacerbated this, with the 'pared down' services requiring women to labour or even give birth alone, with health professionals in PPE. A Covid-safe birth room is unlikely to meet the criteria for romantic sex, let's face it. In spite of this, the data doesn't seem to suggest any great rise in birth interventions,[14] which could be due to a combination of factors – one of which being that the standard birth room was far from optimal pre-Covid, and birth interventions were already extremely high, so although the Covid measures on paper look like they would have made things worse, things can only get so bad.

What does seem to have happened is that women have reported increased levels of anxiety, depression, birth trauma and PTSD. One study of women in England who gave birth during the pandemic found increased levels of distress and anxiety, in particular due to the fluctuating guidance and lack of certainty over whether their partner could be there.[15] The study stated that 46.9 per cent of participants reported that their birth experience was 'predominantly negative'. Another study of UK women found that the prevalence of anxiety and depression had increased under Covid by 60 per cent and 47 per cent respectively, potentially affecting their bond with their baby.[16] A third study, of women in the US, compared their participants to those who gave birth before the pandemic, and found that mothers who gave birth during Covid restrictions were more likely to report postnatal anxiety and PTSD, and have more difficulties with bonding and breastfeeding.[17] In the UK, the Birth Trauma Association reported a big increase in those contacting their support inbox, with numbers roughly tripling between 2020 and 2021.[18]

Within the NHS, the pandemic compounded an already existing problem of underfunding and understaffing in maternity care – the so-called 'midwife crisis'. For every thirty new midwives trained, twenty-nine leave the profession,[19] citing burnout, an inability to provide safe care and disillusionment with a job in which they feel overstretched, taken for granted, and unable to form meaningful relationships with the women they care for.[20] The Royal College of Midwives chief executive Gill Walton has appealed to the government for more funding, describing how maternity services are 'bottom of the list for investment'.[21]

The picture is bleak, and we have certainly drifted a long way from the nurturing birth rooms of the middle ages, a busy, all-female and celebratory affair. In spite of campaigners calling for more humanised, relationship-based care for decades now, birth seems to be only going one way – towards a highly controlled, technologised model, with ever rising rates of induction and caesarean compounded further by midwife shortages and a global pandemic. The March 2022 Ockenden report found serious safety failings in staffing, policies and procedures in UK maternity care,[22] but in the media, articles continue to oversimplify the problems with headlines like 'Three hundred babies lost to a fixation on natural births'.[23] Underneath these stories pervades the deeply held distrust in the female body, and the strong belief that – perhaps like women themselves – it is in need of constant management and monitoring.

In tough times, it is so often women who find themselves being leaned on, their generosity and ability to compensate and 'pick up the slack' exploited. It is so often women who are expected to bend, yield, adapt and have their boundaries transgressed without complaint. It's been well documented that women have been disproportionately affected by the pandemic, for example our livelihood or career plans – and subsequently our mental health – as the default parent for 'home schooling'.[24, 25, 26, 27] Maternity is yet another example of an area in which women's needs have been sidelined with even less apology than usual, and which we are expected to accept without complaint.

## Tracing the origins

I was already in the early stages of writing *Give Birth like a Feminist* in February 2018 when I attended a workshop with Jane Hardwicke Collings about menstruation. Jane runs the School of Shamanic Womancraft in Australia and specialises in teaching what she refers to as 'women's mysteries'. That day spent with her, during her visit to the UK, planted seeds of ideas in my mind about the links between menstruation and birth that I was eventually to come back to during lockdown, when I was asked if I'd be interested in writing a book for preteen girls about periods.

One of Jane's key messages is that when we set up antenatal courses or even write books to guide women through birth preparation, we are catching them too late. They've already been given a decade or two of negative messaging about what their female bodies are capable of, and all of this starts with what we teach them age nine or ten about 'menarche', or the first period. So often this education is laden with shame and negativity, and interlaced with the idea that our bodies are something rather leaky, unpleasant or even disgusting. Many of us carry an entire collection of negative beliefs about our female bodies, perhaps without even realising it – so pervasive and unchallenged is the messaging. Just like with birth, we become the 'fish who can't see the water'. And many of us were passed these beliefs by our mothers, who in turn were passed them by their mothers, and back and back through what is sometimes called our 'mother line' or 'red thread'.

Jane has given me permission to share the questions she asks her workshop attendees. On her behalf, I invite you to consider your own responses. You might like to write down some thoughts about each question, or do this exercise with a female friend, asking each other the questions and discussing them together. What emerges might surprise you.

- What is the story of your own birth? (Include any information about your conception, your mother's pregnancy with you and her/your postnatal experience, as sometimes these times as well as your actual birth can hold important clues for you.)

- How do the women in your family give birth?
- Can you see a connection between how you were born and your menarche (first period)? Note down the story of your first period, or anything you can remember about this transition time in your life: how was it spoken about and taught to you? How did you feel about it? How was it celebrated or not celebrated?
- Can you see any connections between your own birth, your first period, and your overall experience of menstruation?
- Can you see a connection between all of this and how you feel about giving birth/your births if you have already had a baby?
- Can you see a theme or repeating pattern?
- What is arising in your life right now that connects with that?

For many people, there will be themes of shame in these stories. There will almost certainly be situations, going back through the women in your life, in which stories remained forever untold, secrets were kept, or big feelings like grief or anger were never fully expressed. In my own family history, my mother had a miscarriage that was brushed aside and never discussed by my grandmother. At first sight, the story of how she failed to offer my mother a single word of comfort even in the immediate aftermath sounds completely heartless. But unpick the story further, and consider that my grandmother had grown up in a house where her own mother – my great-grandmother – had a series of miscarriages, and lost a child aged two, and you begin to get more of a sense of intergenerational trauma, loss and unspoken grief. And perhaps she had other stories too, which we will never discover, but that made it impossible for her to show warmth or love without reservation. How did my mother then overcome this inheritance of sadness and emotional disconnection when it came to her turn to relate to her own daughter – me? And what of this legacy remains in the way that I mother my own daughters? Something about these experiences of the women in our line gets passed on, even if they happened before our own birth or were never spoken about.

At a more day-to-day level, there will be times in the line of women in our family when basic information was not clearly passed on, simply because of embarrassment or an inability to speak certain words aloud, or name particular body parts or processes. This lack of knowledge about female bodies is not confined to the history books: in a recent survey, only 9 per cent of Britons could label all parts of the vulva, 37 per cent mislabelled the clitoris, and less than half (46 per cent) knew that women have three holes.[28] In another recent survey, almost half of women didn't know where their cervix was.[29]

In the same survey, one in four women misidentified the vagina on a diagram, and although it's not clear if they were asked to label the vulva as part of the same exercise, I would expect that the numbers of women who can't label the vulva or who think the vulva is their 'vagina' would be very high. One survey from Bodyform in 2019 found that 73 per cent of women were confused about what a vulva was.[30] If you're reading this and are also confused, your vagina is the strong and stretchy tube INSIDE YOU that leads from your vulva up to your cervix and uterus; your vulva is all the parts on the OUTSIDE. As I say to my daughters, 'Cup your hand, place it between your legs – everything your hand is touching is your vulva.'

As a mum who uses the word vulva in front of my kids, I'm in a minority: a 2019 survey by the Eve Appeal found that as few as 1 per cent of parents use the word, with less than a fifth using vagina, and nearly half (44 per cent) choosing euphemisms such as 'tuppence', 'front bottom' and 'flower'.[31] These peculiar choices only serve to bake in yet more intergenerational shame – and this has real-world consequences when adult women are too embarrassed to name parts of their own body or seek help for gynaecologial health issues.

# Same bodies, different stories

In writing *My Period*, I wanted to bring alternative ways of presenting young girls with knowledge and information about their bodies into the mainstream. I wanted to give nine-year-old readers a very different sense of their anatomy so that, just like Jane Hardwicke Collings suggested, they turned up to give birth age thirty with a real sense of their female power. A book can be disruptive in this sense, it can offer a shift in perspective – and even the diagrams matter.

I knew there would be diagrams in *My Period*, and I knew I didn't want them all to be 'disembodied'. I was already very familiar with the way in which news outlets so often use faceless photos of 'bumps' to accompany any story about pregnancy or birth. Depicting pregnant women in this way is part of the narrative that does not see a pregnant woman as a whole person, but instead just a 'container' or 'vessel'. The photos don't tell us, 'This article is about a whole person,' but instead present us with a faceless, dehumanised bump. I did not want lots of disembodied uteruses and vulvas in *My Period* for the same reason. Women are whole people, not body parts.

So one day my then ten-year-old daughter came down to find me at the kitchen table trying to use my limited art skills to draw a uterus diagram that somehow included the woman whose uterus was about to be labelled. Inspired by my explanation of why I was doing this, she got out a pencil and did her own sketch – a version of which was eventually adopted by the illustrator, making it into the book. Age ten, it was immediately obvious to my daughter why humanising the illustration was important. Together, in a small way, we had changed the narrative.

I discovered another narrative in need of a rebrand when researching ovulation for the book. Let me place a bet: when you were taught about conception in school, you were shown pictures or maybe a video telling you the story of how the sperm all have a race to get to the egg, and that the best and strongest sperm is the 'winner'?! If you search Google for cartoon images of sperm and egg, you will find the 'winning' sperm wearing sunglasses, in a superhero cape, flexing its biceps, and even offering the egg a bunch of flowers, and you might have been shown this sort of cartoon in school as well.

But what does the egg do in this story? Well, she just sits there and waits. She's portrayed in the cartoons with lipstick, long eyelashes, often blushing and looking with dewy eyes at Mr Hero

Sperm. What nobody tells you, though, is how that particular egg ended up there, rather than any of the others. Your ovaries contain little sacs called follicles where there are always eggs in different stages of development. Each month, some of these eggs start to get bigger and stronger, ready to be released. The 'winning' egg is usually the biggest and strongest, and is released to travel down the fallopian tube.

You could see the egg as a very active player in the story, or even muscly and competitive – or you could at least spin the story that way if it suited your perception of the world. In reality, of course, neither sperm nor egg have a consciousness, or ambition, or any of our cultural understanding of gender (nor do they have sunglasses or eyelashes). But in the story we teach our children, they do, and this says something about the way gender stereotypes are even woven into the stories we present as facts about biology, and the stories we teach our children about their bodies, and the way their bodies are expected to behave.

In trying to research a book about periods I discovered many gaps in my own knowledge of my body, as well as in other women's knowledge of their bodies, and in the collective 'common knowledge' of female biology. Much of what women report as cast-iron fact, like 'when I live with other women our periods synch up' or 'I have more energy when I ovulate', is difficult to corroborate with evidence, as our bodies are extraordinarily underresearched. The gaps are confounded by a lack of basic knowledge; for example, many women may not realise that if they are taking the contraceptive pill, they don't ovulate and therefore don't technically have a 'cycle'. Then there are some areas that seem to be a mystery to everyone, as I found out on several occasions during the writing process, most notably when I tried to discover what 'cervical fluid' actually is, where it's made and how, by what, and from what? I still don't know the answer.

## Invisible powers

Most of us are now familiar with the idea of the so-called 'gender health gap' – the disparity between the way men and women are treated in every area of the health system. This particularly affects research as it creates a 'data gap', placed brilliantly into the spotlight by Caroline Criado Perez in *Invisible Women*. Criado Perez highlights how, with our focus consistently on the male body as the 'default', we are failing to collect data on females in every area from heart attacks to car and seat-belt design. Women suffer in multiple ways as a result – although we have fewer car accidents, for example, when we do, we are much more likely to die or be seriously injured in them, but there is still no 'female' crash test dummy, only a 'scaled-down male' one. Almost all aspects of our world are built by men with men in mind. I think of Criado Perez every time I struggle at the gym to lift the kettle bells, not because they are too heavy, but because the handle width is too big for my hands.

The data gap is detrimental to women in all areas of life, but in areas that only affect women, such as menstruation, pregnancy and birth, it's even worse. These areas are often not studied or investigated at all. Criado Perez touches on childbirth when she writes about the lack of research into the use of oxytocin to augment labour, and tells the story of her friend who had a caesarean because she did not progress past 4cm dilated. 'The experience left her traumatised,' she writes. 'She had flashbacks for the first few weeks after she gave birth. When she talks about the internal exams and procedures, she describes it as a violent assault. But what if it didn't have to be this way?' *Yes,* I thought as I read this sentence. Finally! But Perez goes on, 'What if they'd known from the beginning that she was going to need a caesarean?' Disappointingly, Perez herself seems to me to have a gap here. As so many people do, she's making the assumption that some women just won't progress through labour and reach the required dilation, and that, while this is currently assumed to be pot luck, there might even be a way of telling who these rather unlucky women are in advance. She rightly points out that there could be a way of telling which women will respond to augmentation of labour better than others, or ways of augmenting labour more effectively, both of which are worthy of research. But she doesn't rewind the tape back to the part of the labour *before* the woman's dilation stalled, to ask *why* it has happened. She doesn't ask whether there is something we are doing to women in labour that is preventing their progress. She doesn't notice that we are building birth systems and birth rooms with gaps in our knowledge about female physiology, and that, worse still, nobody seems to care enough about women's birth experiences to address this.

And we could wind the tape back further, to before the labour started, and further still, to the antenatal preparation, and then even further still, to the disembodied bump pics or the passive egg or the period shame or the million and one other subtle messages a woman has received over her lifetime that her body is not only secondary to the male default, but that it's something to apologise for, hide or be ashamed of, rather than something strong and well built that can be trusted or relied upon.

Women were just starting to challenge this. Social media, as you have read elsewhere in this book, has been instrumental in providing a platform for women to talk about their unique female experiences in a way never before possible. From breastfeeding, to menstruation, to miscarriage, to abortion, to endometriosis, to birth, to orgasm, to body hair, women have shared their innermost thoughts and feelings about every single experience imaginable. Their images have been censored and taken down, they have protested, and the images have, perhaps reluctantly, been reinstated. This outpouring of truth has had a direct positive impact, allowing women to share knowledge of these areas of our lives that for so long have been unspoken, shameful and taboo.

Something was being reclaimed. And yet – perhaps a complete coincidence, perhaps not – a new kind of censorship has emerged, one which has us watching our words around the topic of women's bodies again.

## 'Uniquely female experiences'

Phrases like 'women's bodies' or 'uniquely female experiences' have in recent times become complex, in a world that now debates the question of what 'woman' means and who can be included in the definition. In fact, even the way that I have used the word 'woman' throughout this book about childbirth has, since the time of the first publication, become increasingly controversial. Many birth, breastfeeding and menstruation organisations and experts will now replace the word 'woman' with words like 'birthing person', 'lactating parent', 'menstruator' or 'bleeder'. Some will use 'additive language', for example, talking about 'women and birthing people', because 'not all people who birth are women', but this often gets reduced in tweets and Instagram tiles to 'birthing people'.

These changes are due to an ideological shift, which asserts that a person's gender identity – their sense of who they are[32] – holds more importance than their biological sex. Some go further and disregard the concept of biological sex entirely, asserting that there are more than two sexes or that 'sex is a spectrum'.[33, 34] Under this new way of thinking, anyone can be any sex they say they are: a man with a beard and a penis may be a woman and have access to women's spaces and services. 'Not all people who birth are women' means 'a man can give birth'. And 'man' in this context means a person with female biology (otherwise they could not give birth), but who feels themselves to be a man or male. As Kirrin Medcalf, head of trans inclusion for Stonewall, put it at the tribunal of Allison Bailey in 2022, 'Bodies are not inherently male or female.'

Like many of us, the awareness of the effect of gender ideology on the language of childbirth crept onto my radar very slowly and gradually. When I've retraced my steps through my thought processes I've noticed that initially, my own opinion was very often clouded by other people's misogyny and ageism – as women speaking out for women's language and women's rights are so often portrayed, at best, as old and therefore out of touch, at worst, as hateful and bigoted. Rushing through a busy life, I've often accepted this narrative at face value and failed to question it – not realising of course that it would eventually come to be used against me. Now I try much harder to make it my habit to consciously notice when women are being discredited in this way – on any topic – and to try to listen to what *they* are actually saying, rather than what others are saying about them.

The first time I noticed a discussion about sex and gender in the world of childbirth was in 2015. Ina May Gaskin, the world-famous midwife from The Farm in Tennessee (see pages 132–133) signed an open letter to the Midwives Alliance of North America (MANA), along with over 200 other midwives and workers from the field of birth.[35] The letter expressed concern that the word 'woman' had been erased from MANA's 'Core Competencies' document and been replaced with 'pregnant individual' and 'birthing parent'.

The letter applauds MANA for their attempts at inclusivity but raises concerns about 'prioritising gender identity above biological reality', which the letter authors see as part of a cultural trend to 'deny material biological reality and further disconnect ourselves from nature and the body'. They state: 'The root of female oppression is derived from biology', and also point out, 'Women have a right to bodily autonomy and to speak about their bodies and lives without the demand that we couch this self-expression in language which suits the agenda of others who were not born female.'

They don't just talk about female biology as the root of our oppression, but also affirm it as our 'life-giving power' – perhaps not surprising from a group made up entirely of midwives. If women are erased from the language of birth, they argue, 'women as a class lose recognition of and connection to this power'.

I remember skimming through the letter at the time and not fully understanding what they were trying to say. Why were they objecting to more inclusive language? I had always held inclusivity to be an unequivocally positive thing, and was surprised that such a large group of female birth workers – not usually a group renowned for unkindness or bigotry – seemed to be arguing so passionately against it. Any attempt I may have made to unravel this seeming contradiction was soon drowned out by the dominant narrative that Ina May Gaskin was a 'transphobe'.

With that incident largely forgotten, I went on to write *The Positive Birth Book*, published in 2017, and this one, published in 2019. In the two years between those books there was a shift in the UK world of birth and maternity, towards the use of the term 'birthing people' or 'women and birthing people'. When writing *Give Birth like a Feminist*, I debated at length whether or not to use the phrase, or to write some kind of 'disclaimer' at the front of the book as to what I meant by the word 'woman' – I'd seen others do this. But something nagged at me. Maybe I'd taken in more of the MANA letter than I thought. I eventually decided that a book about sex-based oppression – a book about how women are basically kept from the power of their own biology by a maternity system built by the patriarchy – ought to use sex-based language. I stuck to 'woman' and thankfully nobody seemed to object.

While writing *Give Birth like a Feminist* I also began to read more about 'gender-critical' feminism, in part because an academic paper about obstetric violence that I read as part of my research cited a UK paper about the polarised interpretations of the medicalisation of childbirth, written by the feminist philosopher Jane Clare Jones.[36] I chatted to Jane briefly and began following her on Twitter, initially completely ignorant to the fact that Jane was a leading radical feminist voice, already fully embroiled in the discussion about gender ideology. Her tweets on the issue were prolific, and insightful. Jane's voice gave me a window into a different perspective, outside the world of midwives and doulas, many of whom seemed very willing to change their language when talking about women's bodies. Many, but not all. Lynsey McCarthy-Calvert took a stand in 2019 that ended with her being forced to step down as spokesperson for Doula UK. Responding on social media to a reference by Cancer Research UK to 'everyone with a cervix', Lynsey wrote: 'I am not a "cervix owner", I am not a "menstruator". I am not a "feeling". I am not defined by wearing a dress and lipstick. I am a woman: an adult human female. Women birth all the people, make up half the population, but less than a third of the seats in the House of Commons are occupied by us.' While Lynsey's point was centred on holding the boundaries around the material reality of being female, the prevailing response was that she was bigoted, transphobic, unkind, out of touch. An article from *Pink News* drew a line of association from Lynsey all the way to white nationalist extremists. She was ostracised by the birth world and most people remained silent, presumably worried that if they defended her they would be subject to the same fate.

As I became more curious about all of this, 2020 happened. During the lockdowns that followed I started to read everything I could find about 'gender'. I wanted to understand the origin of phrases such 'birthing people', and 'assigned female or male at birth'. I asked these questions in birth and midwifery groups: 'Who decided that the term "birthing people" was acceptable?' 'Where did the idea of sex being "assigned" originate?' 'Surely a baby's sex is observed, not at birth, but in utero, at the scan, isn't it?' and every time I did, I was quickly told my questions were transphobic and even, on one occasion, asked to leave a group completely. The fact that these basic questions did not seem to be acceptable only spurred me on and made me ever more curious. What happened next, some of you may have read about. In November 2020, I was tagged in an Instagram post about obstetric violence on the International Day to End Violence Against Women. One of the slides in the post read:

> *Obstetric violence is about power and patriarchy.*
> *Birthing people are seen as the 'fragile sex' who need to*
> *be kept under patriarchal authority by doctors.*

Having written a book about the sex-based nature of disrespectful maternity care, I felt this statement needed to be challenged. The patriarchal authority they mention indeed exists, but it's not exercised over 'people', it's exercised specifically over females: women. And so I responded with: 'It is women who are seen as the "fragile sex" etc, and obstetric violence is violence against women. Let's not forget who the oppressed are here, and why.'

And then, all hell broke loose. In what can only be described as a social media bin fire, I was called 'violent', 'a piece of shit', 'TERF', 'toxic', 'dangerous', a 'vile creature', 'wilfully harmful' and much, much more. There were calls to throw my books in the bin. A breastfeeding support worker shared a meme 'How to Give Birth like an Exclusionary White Feminist', writing underneath:

> *Let's just air it. Milli Hill. We shouldn't be buying her books. We shouldn't be gifting them. We shouldn't be following her. We shouldn't be quoting her. She has dangerous opinions, beliefs and views.*

As the bin fire blazed, the charity Birthrights, which I had supported in every way I could for nearly a decade, made a social media post about 'inclusivity' which everyone in the world of maternity could immediately identify as being pointed at me. Later that night, as I sat on my sofa in utter shock at what was happening, I received an email from the CEO of Birthrights, effectively saying that they would no longer associate with me: 'We are unable to work with people who do not share our inclusive values,' they said.

This experience was quite terrifying, and I felt as if my world was suddenly imploding. I spent several months lying low, feeling deeply upset and thinking more about what to do. And then, in June 2021, three things happened at once. Jess de Wahls fought back against her 'cancellation' by the Royal Academy,[37] Chimamanda Ngozi Adichie published her essay 'It Is Obscene',[38] and Maya Forstater won her appeal, establishing in law that believing that 'humans cannot change sex' is a protected belief under the Equality Act 2010.[39] At this point I felt like this was a conversation I wanted to be a part of. What had happened to me felt relevant to the wider discussion, not just about gender, but also about the way in which women were being punished if they ask questions or challenge the direction of travel. I wrote a long blog post about my experiences, entitled, 'I will not be silenced', and published it in July 2021. That week my story was covered in various newspapers, and J.K. Rowling tweeted to support me. The relief of finally speaking my mind and not worrying about the backlash as a result was . . . well, let's just say it was extremely therapeutic. Since then, the conversation around gender has continued to open up in a way that was unimaginable just a year or so ago. People have begun to understand that there are conflicts of rights when we accept that 'anyone who says they are a woman is literally a woman'. We can see this illustrated starkly in sports, for example, as with trans woman Lia Thomas competing in the women's category of swimming, moving from the mid-500s in the men's ranking to being a top-ranked swimmer in the women's category.[40] But there are other areas of concern; for example, women-only spaces like domestic violence refuges, prisons and hospital wards and women-only shortlists and panels, along with data and research. We are a long way from resolving all this, but we have at least moved on from the somewhat chilling concept of 'no debate'.

For a while, I was slightly baffled as to why I had ended up in this whole situation. Surely the topics I write about – birth, breastfeeding, motherhood and periods – are a million miles away from issues around gender, and being trans. It took me a while to understand that it is precisely the material reality of these 'uniquely female experiences' that is standing in the way of a movement that wishes to make 'woman' an open category. Unless you uncouple the concept of 'woman' from 'female biology', male people cannot ever truly be women. When you think about it like this, you can see precisely why I ended up in the firing line.

# The desexing of language

In spite of the fact that it would certainly have made for a much easier life, I have reflected and read and reflected and questioned some more and I cannot in good conscience detach 'woman' from the reality of biological sex. There is much confusion in the current debate between the meanings of 'sex' and 'gender'. I think it's important to always be clear that when I use the word 'woman', I am using it in its sexed sense, to mean a female person. Women are oppressed and discriminated against on the basis of their sex, and to fight this sex-based oppression, we need sex-based language. In this sexed sense, for example, it is not 'birthing people' who are seen as 'the fragile sex', or as 'vessels', disposable containers for the next generation whose feelings and experiences are secondary. It is women. The oppression of women in childbirth, and in *particular* obstetric violence, happens to women, not because of their gender identity, but because of their sex. As in so many other situations, denying this biological reality, and taking away the words to describe it, will only enable it to go unchallenged.

This has recently been explored by a group of academics in a paper entitled 'Effective communication about pregnancy, birth, lactation, breastfeeding and newborn care: The importance of sexed language'.[41] The authors, a global team of women's health experts, warn that while desexing the language of female reproduction is done with the intent of being kind, 'this kindness has delivered unintended consequences that have serious implications for women and children'. Among many examples, they cite the September 2021 front cover of the world-renowned *Lancet* journal, which referred to women as 'bodies with vaginas'. They demonstrate this is part of a wider trend to remove sexed terms such as 'women' and 'mothers' from discussions about female reproduction – a trend that may be born of good intentions but without consideration of the possible consequences.

When women hear 'inclusive terminology' they very often object because they find it immediately dehumanising – we instinctively don't want to be called 'birthing bodies' or 'cervix-havers' or 'non-men'. The paper authors agree – and mention the long history of the medical profession sidelining and dismissing women's bodies as faulty and treating the male body as standard. This language, they say, threatens to unravel decades of work in improving the visibility of women in medicine. Added to this, they argue, instead of being inclusive, the new terminology risks excluding some women, in particular those who are young or who have low literacy or education, or those who are not reading information in their first language. In a world in which even educated women may not know the location of their cervix, or even if they have one, being referred to as a 'cervix-haver' may actually put them at risk of missing vital health information.

Sex-based language matters when it comes to informing women of their rights, too. It's not the same to talk about 'pregnant families' giving informed consent in labour, which implies that people other than the woman are entitled to make choices about what happens to her body, when so many people (myself included) have been striving for the opposite – clear autonomy for the woman in labour. Furthermore, say the researchers, inclusive language can risk obscuring data. If we state that one in twenty people are susceptible to a particular medical condition, this is a different statistic to suggesting one in twenty *women* are susceptible. This was well illustrated during the pandemic when the Australian Government Department of Health and Aged Care changed an information leaflet, which initially read:

> **Pregnant women** *with COVID-19 have a higher risk of certain complications compared to* **non-pregnant women** *with COVID-19.*

In between June and August 2021 this was updated to read:

> **Pregnant people** *with COVID-19 have a higher risk of certain complications compared to* **non-pregnant people** *with COVID-19.*

This obscures the data because a non-pregnant person can of course be male, so 'non-pregnant people' refers to the entire population who are not pregnant. And although the document was then amended again, the version with the data obscured was copied and distributed by South Australia Health, and the error introduced by the desexed language was spread. It does make you wonder why it would be decided that removing references to 'woman' is important enough to risk obscuring vital health messaging.

The prevailing narrative has been that there is absolutely nothing to lose and everything to gain from so-called 'additive language', but the authors of the new paper have clearly set out the precise ways in which these changes can be detrimental. As well as being dehumanising and obscuring health messages, desexed language could also undermine breastfeeding, they say, for example by disembodying it and making this 'human milk' sound like something separate to the mother. The paper's authors also argue that if we lose the word 'mother', we lose something bigger than the word. It's a word that holds meaning beyond 'parent'; it's the first word that most infants will say, and perhaps the oldest word ever spoken. Do we really want to replace it, and potentially risk losing all of the nurture and connection that is associated with it too?

There has been pushback against the desexing of language from other areas. In November 2021 the charity British Pregnancy Advisory Service (BPAS) put out a strategy document in which they explained why they felt it important to continue to use the word 'woman' in their services.[42] They wrote:

*Women's reproductive healthcare and choices
remain regulated and restricted in the way they are
precisely because they are women's issues, sadly still
bound up with heavily gendered and judgmental
approaches to female sexuality, ideals of motherhood
and expectations of maternal sacrifice, and the need
to control women's bodies and choices. If we cannot
clearly articulate that it is predominantly women,
rather than people at large, who are affected by this
we will find it much harder to dismantle a framework
that today is still underpinned by sexism, and achieve
a broader goal of ensuring that everyone, no matter
how they identify, can access the care and support they
need as swiftly and straightforwardly as possible.*

Making a statement such as this is not without controversy – 200 people signed a letter against the BPAS statement,[43] while 1,743 signed an open letter to support their stance.[44] It's noteworthy that there does not seem to be the same pressure for language changes in the area of men's health. The charity Prostate Cancer UK, for example, use the hashtag #MenWeAreWithYou and in October 2021, when challenged about their repeated use of the word 'men' on Twitter, they replied, 'We are of course aware that trans women have prostates, however we want to reach as many at-risk individuals as possible and have chosen to use the word men to achieve this.'

# Spare ribs

There's a photo that does the rounds from time to time on social media, showing a woman at a protest – I wish I knew who or where she was – grinning and holding a placard that bears the words, 'I didn't come from your rib, you came from my vagina'. After the belly laugh it induces, we can contemplate what's underneath – a neat challenge to the androcentric narrative that sidelines women's power and continues to insist that men come first and foremost.

This is the narrative that was played out in the pandemic, when women took the career hit of home education during lockdowns and when birth experiences took the hit of being 'pared back to what was essential' – crucial to the system, but not to women themselves. This is the narrative that has led to decades of research focused on the male body as standard with little effort made to understand women's health. This is the narrative that leads to birth rooms built with flagrant disregard to female physiology, by a system that continues to shrug when women are damaged by poor care and birth trauma. This is the narrative that tells us our bodies are at best a mystery, and at worst a mistake, and that teaches us even from our first period that being female is something we must endure rather than celebrate. And this is the narrative that tells us that our words – the very linguistic form we give to our selves, our biology, our sex-based rights, our experiences and our existence – are disposable or even offensive and must be adjusted or lost to accommodate and make room for the needs of others.

Women are not a second thought after the male default. We are people in our own right, and our biology holds power and sets us apart. In the birth room we face a choice, to accept the prevailing narrative or to challenge it. In a world where women's rights are currently under threat – for example in the USA where abortion rights are being reversed – it has never been more important for women to challenge, to take up space, to refuse to be sidelined, to defend our sex-based rights and to assert that, as whole people, we matter. A healthy baby is not all that matters. Women matter too.

# Stand and Deliver

## A letter to pregnant readers

Knowledge brings power, for sure, but, 'with great power, comes great responsibility'. Apparently that's a quote from *Spiderman*, but it sounds pretty weighty, so I'm going to steal it.

In your birth, you may not want to be the superhero, if doing so means that you have to have all the responsibility. Reading this book may have made you feel worried that, in order to 'qualify' as a feminist, you have to somehow take charge in birth and become more skilled and better informed than even the professionals attending you. I want to reassure you that this is not the case. What this book is aiming for is a new landscape for birth, in which power and respect flow mutually between midwives, doctors and the women in their care. For this to happen, yes, women do need to take some responsibility for their birth – some, but not all. There will be times when you want to hold on to your power tightly, and times when you want to hand it over, willingly and urgently. The key, perhaps, is that you decide, and that your power is given, not taken.

This book has urged you to challenge and reconsider everything you thought you knew about childbirth. It has asked you to think about the way we talk about our birth choices and about the imbalanced power dynamic embedded in phrases like 'I am not allowed', and 'all that matters is a healthy baby'. It has suggested that birth is an overlooked feminist issue, and that we urgently need to shine the harsh spotlight of #metoo into the labour ward, even if this raises tough questions about how we approach a uniquely female experience in a world where the feminist fight has been largely focused on equality. We've travelled back in time to explore the historical events that have led us to where we are now – a world in which we know a great deal about what women need in birth and yet so many of us don't seem to be getting it. As I make the finishing touches to this book, the 2018 Care Quality Commission report has been published, highlighting, among other things, that only 15 per cent of UK women who gave birth last year knew the midwife who attended them in labour, and that 36 per cent of them gave birth 'lying with their feet in stirrups'.

With the idea in mind that how we 'do' birth is a symptom of our age, I've asked you to contemplate how history will judge our current approach. All of us are trying to loosen the grip that technology has on us – drawing us away from family, relationships, and nature, and into a place where we look at screens more than we look at faces – and at the same time we all want to keep the many benefits that medical and technological advances have brought us. This book has suggested that we can, and we must, have both age-old human connection *and* twenty-first-century technology available to us in our births. And at the moment, in the Western world, a technologised birth is becoming increasingly more common, and a humanised birth harder and harder to come by. As women, and feminists, and as the ones who actually have to 'do' the birthing, we need to challenge this trend.

As we have also seen, being 'challenging' about how, where and with whom we birth can have us labelled as 'unrealistic', 'difficult', or even 'bad mothers' or 'mad'. Just as society has a history of strict guidelines around women's sexual behaviour, so too are we expected to birth in ways that are compliant, passive and serve the needs of others over our own. This compliance is perpetuated by fear and misinformation – we are taught that our female bodies are not built to give birth well, and we therefore readily accept the help we think we need. Ironically, the 'help' we are offered is in itself built on a poor understanding of female physiology, but when it hinders us more than it actually assists, we are encouraged to think that our bodies did indeed let us down. This book has asked you to think about how the culture that surrounds you props up this status quo, from the beliefs you may unquestioningly hold about the shape of your pelvis, to the sterile births of *One Born Every Minute*, and about how true knowledge could potentially break these negative loops.

Finally, we've had a whistle-stop tour of human rights in childbirth. Was it a revelation to you, as it is to so many, to discover that you have some of these rights? The fact that your answer is most probably yes makes me glad that I wrote this book and that you read it, even if it's been tough at times or made you or those who are charged with your maternity care feel uncomfortable. Change is not a comfortable process: ask a caterpillar about that. And in the long history of humankind, nobody has ever been handed their rights on a plate. Progress in human rights always begins with noticing your particular oppression. It then always, *always* involves a situation in which those rights are asked for, demanded and consistently denied. The person or group asking for their rights will be portrayed as wrong, irresponsible, angry, aggressive, destructive, ill-informed and mad. Rights are never willingly given. They always have to be fought for, they always have to be claimed.

Every individual reading this book can be part of this change. If you are in a role that allows you to 'pull strings' in terms of the finance, direction or structure of maternity care, ask yourself how you can contribute to a maternity system that is truly respectful of the process of childbirth as both a physiological function and a psycho-spiritual rite of passage. Don't be afraid to think of birth in those terms, because if we can't acknowledge that the moment a new life begins deserves some reverence, then it's probably time to admit that this whole humanity thing is pointless and overrated. So – what strings can you pull to bring beauty and human connection and soul into these birthing moments? Whether you green-light the new black-out blinds for the birth centre, or roll out nationwide woman-centred policies, you can make a difference to individual women's memories of birth that will last a lifetime.

And if you are a health care professional, midwife or doctor, it goes without saying that you can be part of the change. You can spend some time thinking about the part you play in the drama of the modern birth room, and challenge your own views and assumptions about how birth 'is' and how birth 'can be'. You can work towards more personalised, individualised care, with more eye contact and less screen contact. You can talk with your colleagues, openly and honestly, and you can check up on your personal biases and on your privilege and how this may cloud your perspective. Most importantly, you can raise your empathy game, asking yourself on a moment-by-moment basis how the women in your care actually *feel*. If that last bit annoyed you or made you feel defensive, bingo: you are not currently doing this enough. If you're really mad at me now and absolutely insistent you are the most empathic practitioner you can be, then – keep doing what you are doing. I believe you.

But I'm not talking to commissioners, politicians or obstetricians in this book, although I hope they are reading and listening in. I'm talking to women who birth: those who are pregnant, those who have had one baby and might have another, those who are hopeful to be mothers one day. You are the ones who have to actually perform the seemingly impossible, mind-bendingly miraculous, utterly everyday task of bringing a new human into the world, out of your very own body. You are the ones who deserve the best possible chance to enter the tunnel of labour or birth feeling tough and supported, and emerge the other side feeling triumphant, powerful, ecstatic, energised, proud and full of confidence in your abilities. You are the ones I care about, whose birth stories keep driving me to repeat the mantras: *birth is a feminist issue, birth can be different, birth can be better, women matter too.* And no, you cannot shoulder all of the responsibility to improve birth, or even to improve your own birth. Women may have superpowers, but change often happens painfully slowly, and it may take years or even generations to turn birth around and get it back onto a course that truly serves every woman as an individual. But you, you are where this change starts. The change starts with you. Here's what you can do.

## Be an adult

Refuse to be infantilised, patronised or mansplained in your maternity care. Behave in the same strong grown-up way that you behave in other areas of your life, such as your career or your relationship. Watch out for signs that your status is shifting away from 'woman' and towards 'girl' – this might be signs from you such as feeling small, not feeling heard, feeling petulant, feeling like you are 'being naughty' – or want to be. Or it might be signs from others that they are trying to place you in this role, such as calling you a 'good girl', talking to you in a stern or infantilising way, or placating you with trivialities such as 'this will all soon be over'. If you feel this happening, try to centre yourself and remind yourself that you are a grown-up. Demand proper explanations, ask for evidence, ask to have risks and benefits clearly explained, and, if necessary, remind others of your human right to be the key decision maker in the birth process. Vote with your feet if you need to and change care provider – even during labour you can ask to be attended by somebody different. Remind yourself that it is OK to be clear, strong and determined in your maternity care – in other words, stand up for yourself – just as you do in other areas of your life.

## Know you matter

You are important, and your experience of birth is important. Refuse to let what you want and need be sidelined, minimalised or dismissed. Caring about yourself does not mean you care less about your baby. It goes without saying that you have the safety and best interest of your baby at the heart of everything you do. That's a given – but what else matters? This will be different for different women – for example, you need to give birth where and with whom you feel safe, but this won't be the same for everyone. Allow yourself to consider what is truly important to you. Speak these needs aloud. Write them down in a bullet-pointed list. If necessary, laminate it!

## Make plans

Birth plans are not pointless. They are a clear expression of what you want and need – this could only be pointless if you didn't matter, and you do matter. For this reason, be extra wary of the motivations of anyone who insists on telling you that you are wasting your time. Make a plan, discuss it with your care providers, and ask them to document that they have done so. Creating your plan is a process in itself, during which you can consider all your many options and learn about your choices, and your rights. It's a chance to think clearly about what you want to happen in every eventuality, not just in the 'perfect birth' (if such a thing exists!).

Build contingency and secondary plans into your birth plan, and remember that, as an adult, you are well equipped to cope with disappointment if you don't get the birth you want. However, don't be afraid to 'shoot for the moon' – visualising your ideal birth may help you to get it – and as they say, if you miss at least you will be among the stars.

## Challenge the 'language of permission'

Prick up your ears for any time you hear the imbalanced power dynamic of maternity care coming your way in a phrase like 'you are not allowed' or 'they don't let you'. Remember: you *are* allowed. Nobody can tell you what you can or cannot do with your own body, and nobody can do anything to you and your body without your full permission. Knowing this does not mean you have to decline anything and everything or start a war with your care providers. It just means that you get to have that confidence and feeling of safety inside that comes from knowing that you are in the driving seat. If you hear the language of permission, call it out. Help confine this inaccurate way of viewing women's maternity rights to the history books.

## Know there is no right or wrong way to give birth

Giving birth like a feminist means birthing your way, not my way or anybody else's way. Different well-informed women will come to different conclusions about what is the best choice for them. There are no boxes to tick, or points to be given out. Conforming to one set of choices does not mean you qualify to be a certain kind of woman or in a certain kind of club. You can mix your choices up, too – be a formula-feeding, elective-caesarean-choosing stay-at-home-mum or a home-birthing tandem-feeding high-flying city analyst. Refuse to be put into boxes and resist the 'mummy wars' – which are almost certainly driven by the media rather than women themselves. On the whole, women are usually open-minded and supportive of other women's choices – we are all in the mother ship together and there is a certain kind of solidarity that comes from this somewhat wild and intergalactic ride. Drop the guilt – it's your body, your baby and your choice.

## Watch out for polarity

Polarity is a 'Thing' right now. Think politics. Think Trump. Think Brexit. Think pink and blue gender-coded kids. Think veganism, abstinence from alcohol, clean eating; the list goes on. Going to extremes has become the way it's done, and birth has fallen into this trap somewhat. Dialogue about birth tends to become 'birth wars', with the 'your body was made to do this' brigade on one side and the 'take all the drugs' bunch on the other. Beyond these polarities are further extremes: all the medical help going, no medical help at all; freebirth, or elective caesarean, for example. Don't get caught up in this. Be unique. Be an individual, with individual, specific needs. There is room for nuance in your birth choices. There is room for you to make decisions, and then change your mind. Maybe your body was made to do this, but it didn't feel like it on the day. Maybe you thought you were made to do this, but in fact, you did have a genuine health issue that meant modern medicine saved you or your baby's life. Maybe you wanted all the drugs, but in the end you only had a few, or none. Maybe you weren't coping in labour, and then suddenly, you were coping, and then you weren't again. Maybe you hypnobirthed and yelled your head off from beginning to end. Maybe you hated some of it and loved some of it; maybe you were afraid, *and* lost control, *and* totally nailed it. Let birth surprise you – allow it to be complicated, real and human.

## Demand the best care you can get

Relationship-based care from a midwife you know and trust is the gold standard that every woman deserves. Ask for this. Raise your voice and say what's important to you. If you have health complications that mean your care is obstetric led, then relationships are still important, so build them with your doctors, and try to get continuity too. If you cannot get the kind of care you want, keep asking – perhaps there is another way? Can you change to a different trust or hospital? What if you ask for a home birth? Do you have a nearby birth centre? Persist. Doors may open. Either way, consider hiring a doula or, if you have the budget, an independent midwife. If you don't have the budget, get in touch with them anyway, as many have access funds or reduced fees for people on low income. Making conscious choices about your care will improve your chances of having a positive birth experience.

## Think of other women too

Feminist issues need feminist activism. You may not be able to change things for yourself. Perhaps you have already had your babies, or maybe you feel you are banging your head against a brick wall in terms of the lack of choice currently available to you in your local area. Keep going. By asking for things to be different, you are paving the way for a different kind of maternity experience for women of the future. It is only when women ask for the unavailable that providers will begin to see just how many women want the very thing they are failing to offer. It is only when women complain about the care they receive that providers will hear their voices collectively getting louder, and harder to ignore. By saying what you want and don't want in the birth room, and saying it clear and strong, you are doing not just yourself but women of the future a really big favour. That's true feminism.

Finally, remember that while you cannot *control* birth, you can certainly *influence* it. It's OK to try to do this, and it's OK for your birth experience to be important to you. A healthy baby is not *all* that matters. You matter too.

# Resources

The following organisations provide support with birth choices, advocacy and human rights in various global locations. Should you have a specific issue or enquiry, they should also be able to signpost you to support groups in your local area.

**AIMS**
Promoting better births, rights and choice. Helpline & support.
http://www.aims.org.uk/

**AIMS Ireland**
Promoting choices and rights in Ireland
http://aimsireland.ie/about-us/

**Alliance Francophone pour L'Accouchment Respecte (AFAR)**
French advocacy, rights, information and respectful care
https://afar.info

**Aperio**
Humanised birth in Czech Republic
https://www.aperio.cz/

**Associacao Gravidez e Parto**
Human rights and birth choice in Portugal
http://www.associacaogravidezeparto.pt

**Association of Radical Midwives**
Support for pregnant women and midwives including a helpline
https://www.midwifery.org.uk/

**Birthrights**
Promoting respect for human rights in UK birth
http://www.birthrights.org.uk/

**Birth Monopoly**
USA based: working to challenge the imbalance of power
https://birthmonopoly.com/

**El Parto Es Nuestro**
Birth improvement and advocacy in Spain and Latin America
https://www.elpartoesnuestro.es/

**EMMA Egyesulet**
Humanisation of birth in Hungary
http://www.emmaegyesulet.hu/

**Fundacja Rodzic Poludzku**
Respectful maternity care in Poland
https://www.rodzicpoludzku.pl/

**GeboorteBeweging**
Human rights in childbirth in the Netherlands
http://geboortebeweging.nl

**Human Rights In Childbirth**
Promoting human rights in birth globally
http://www.humanrightsinchildbirth.org/

**Improving Birth**
Advocating for evidence based birth in the USA
https://improvingbirth.org/

**Make Birth Better**
Prevention and support of birth trauma in the UK
https://www.makebirthbetter.org/

**Maternity Action**
Employment and working rights for UK pregnant women and parents
https://www.maternityaction.org.uk/

**Maternity Choices Australia**
Leading Australian maternity consumer body
http://www.maternitychoices.org.au/

**Maternity Consumer Network**
Australian membership network to improve birth
https://www.maternityconsumernetwork.org.au/

**Motherhood**
Parent information and advocacy in Germany
https://www.mother-hood.de

**Obstetric Violence Observatory Italy**
Advocacy, support, and data collection on obstetric violence in Italy
https://ovoitalia.wordpress.com

**Positive Birth Movement**
Global network of free antenatal groups linked by social media
http://www.positivebirthmovement.org

**RODA**
Dignity in childbirth in Croatia
http://www.roda.hr/

**Rodilnitza**
Improving birth rights in Bulgaria
http://www.rodilnitza.com

**White Ribbon Alliance**
Demanding the right for a safe and respectful birth globally
http://whiteribbonalliance.org/

# Acknowledgements

This book would not have come into being without large numbers of people. First and foremost, I'd like to thank my agent Jane at Graham Maw Christie, who had utter confidence in me and in the ideas which underpin *Give Birth Like a Feminist* right from the start. Her quiet assurance has gently nurtured the book from seed to fruit. Thanks also to the entire team at HQ for their passion and enthusiasm, and for the skilful and sensitive editing of Kate Fox and Katy Denny. Big gratitude too to editor Rachel Kenny, who originally backed the book, and her gorgeous baby Freddie.

Thanks to everyone who has run, runs, or will run a Positive Birth Movement group. You all do it for free and out of passion for true freedom of choice in birth, and for this I am full of awe and gratitude. You are feminism in action.

So many people have shared their expertise with me, but a particular thanks to my dedicated support squad: Professor Lesley Page CBE (former RCM President), Dr Sheena Byrom OBE (midwife and advocate of humanised birth), Dr Alison Barrett (NZ obstetrician, thinker and writer), Professor Hannah Dahlen (Australian researcher and midwife), Mary Newburn (service user researcher and persistent maternity activist), Natalie Lennard (photographer and creator of Birth Undisturbed), Dr Camilla Pickles (postdoctoral researcher of obstetric violence and the law), Dr Julie Roberts (research fellow, pregnancy and birth in social context), Professor Soo Downe OBE (researcher and globally renowned expert in normal birth), Catherine Williams (evidence expert and former NICE fellow), Jayne Rice-Oxley (specialist in human rights in birth), Dr Elizabeth Newnham (midwife academic) and Michelle Quashie (advocate for women's voices in childbirth).

More love and thanks goes to, in no particular order, Maddie McMahon for her 'book doula-ing' skills; Kay King for her support developing the PBM; Hermine Hayes-Klein for all that she has done for human rights in birth; Cristen Pascucci for her razor-sharp birth activism (America needs you!); Becky Reed for her friendship and insight; all of the wonderful crew I met at the inspirational (and deeply feminist) Home Birth Conference in Sydney: Jo Hunter, Amantha McGuinness, Jerusha Sutton, Lucretia McCarthy, Nadine Fragosa, and Rhea Dempsey; Abigail Blackburn for the great team we made at Best and her friendship; Dr Rachel Reed for her help with my thoughts on induction and 'OASI'; Jane Hardwicke Collings for her amazing insight into menstrual cycles; Duncan and Sue Spencer who let me write several chapters in their peaceful spare room; and Daniela Dran for sharing her knowledge of human rights in birth with me. There are so many other people who have freely given their time and wisdom, in so many ways. I can't mention them all but I am utterly grateful to each and every one of you.

Finally, I'd like to thank my wonderful partner George Litchfield, who has patiently held the space for me while I have birthed three babies and two books, each time feeding me, soothing me, listening to me moan and wail and reassuring me that I would get there in the end. Big love to my mum Pauline Hill, and of course, to my absolutely, totally and utterly gorgeous children, Bess, Ursula and Albie. They have been incredibly supportive of mummy's need to 'get this book done' and I think even a little bit proud of me (perhaps in particular because 'it's the same publisher as David Walliams' and 'you are going to be famous, just like him, mum'). Whilst this might not be quite the case, I do hope I continue to make them proud. They are the reason I get out of bed in the morning, and they make me want to be the best person I can be. For this, I'm eternally grateful.

# Bibliography

*We Should All Be Feminists*, Chimamanda Ngozie Adichie, Fourth
      Estate, 2014

*Immaculate Deception, A New Look at Women and Childbirth*, Suzanne
      Arms, Houghton Mifflin, 1975

*The Handmaid's Tale*, Margaret Atwood, McClelland and Stewart, 1985

*Women and Power*, Mary Beard, Profile Books, 2017

*The Second Sex*, Simone de Beauvoir, Vintage Classics, 1997

*Am I Allowed?*, Beverley A. Lawrence Beech, AIMS, 2014

*Games People Play*, Eric Berne, Grove Press, 1964

*Water Birth Unplugged, Proceedings of the First International Water
      Birth Conference*, ed. Beverley A. Lawrence Beech, Books for
      Midwives, 1996

*How to Heal a Bad Birth, Making Sense, Making Peace and Moving On*,
      Melissa Bruijn and Debby Gould, Birthtalk.org, 2016

*The Roar Behind the Silence, Why Kindness, Compassion and Respect
      Matter in Maternity Care*, ed. Sheena Byrom and Soo Downe,
      Pinter &Martin, 2015

*End of Equality, Manifestos for the* 21st *century*, Beatrix Campbell,
      Seagull Books, 2014

*The Hero with a Thousand Faces*, Joseph Campbell, Fontana Press, 1993

*Birth: A History*, Tina Cassidy, Chatto & Windus, 2007

*Rage Becomes Her, The Power of Women's Anger*, Soraya Chemaly,
      Simon and Schuster UK, 2018

*Herstory: Womanifesto*, Jane Hardwicke Collings, self-published
      pamphlet, 2002

*Do It Like A Woman...and Change the World*, Caroline Criado-Perez, Portobello Books, 2015

*Childbirth and Authoritative Knowledge, Cross-Cultural Perspectives*, ed. Robbie. E. Davis-Floyd and Carolyn F. Sargent, University of California Press, 1997

*Birth with Confidence, Savvy Choices for Normal Birth*, Rhea Dempsey, Boathouse Press, Australia, 2013

*Childbirth Without Fear*, Grantly Dick-Read, Heinemann Medical Books, 1942

*Witches, Midwives and Nurses, A History of Women Healers*, Barbara Ehrenreich and Deidre English, Feminist Press, 1973, Second Edition, 2010

*Birthing from Within, An Extra-ordinary Guide to Childbirth Preparation*, Pam England and Rob Horowitz, Souvenir Press, London 2007

*Like a Mother, a Feminist Journey Through the Science and Culture of Pregnancy*, Angela Garbes, Harper Collins, New York, 2018

*Ina May's Guide to Childbirth*, Ina May Gaskin, Vermilion, 2008

*The Female Eunuch*, Germaine Greer, MacGibbon and Kee Ltd, 1970

*The Whole Woman*, Germaine Greer, Doubleday, 1999

*I'm OK, You're OK*, Thomas A. Harris, Harper, 1967

*Birth and Sex, the Power and the Passion*, Sheila Kitzinger, Pinter & Martin, 2012

*The Experience of Childbirth*, Sheila Kitzinger, Victor Gollancz, 1962

*Rediscovering Birth*, Sheila Kitzinger, Little, Brown, 2000

*On Becoming a Mother*, Brigid McConville, Oneworld, 2014

*How to Be a Woman*, Caitlin Moran, Ebury Press, 2011

*Reading Birth and Death, a History of Obstetric Thinking*, Jo Murphy-Lawless, Cork University Press, 1998

*Towards the Humanization of Birth: A Study of Epidural Analgesia and Hospital Birth Culture*, Elizabeth Newnham, Lois McKellar, Jan Pincombe, Palgrave Macmillan, 2018

*Burning Woman*, Lucy H. Pearce, Womancraft Publishing, Cork, 2016

*The Politics of the Body*, Alison Phipps, Polity Press, 2014

*Why Induction Matters*, Rachel Reed, Pinter & Martin, 2018

*Of Woman Born*, Adrienne Rich, Virago, 1977

*Why Human Rights in Childbirth Matter*, Rebecca Schiller, 2016

*When Survivors Give Birth, Understanding and Healing the Effects of Early Sexual Abuse on Childbearing Women*, Penny Simkin, Phyllis Klaus, Classic Day Publishing, 2004

*Men Explain Things to Me*, Rebecca Solnit, Haymarket Books, 2014

*Pregnancy, Birth and Maternity Care, Feminist Perspectives*, ed. Mary Stewart, Books for Midwives/Elsevier, 2004

*Misconceptions*, Naomi Wolf, Chatto & Windus, 2001

*Vagina, a New Biography*, Naomi Wolf, Virago, 2012

*A Vindication of the Rights of Woman*, Mary Wollstonecraft, 1792

# Endnotes

## INTRODUCTION

1    'Making childbirth a positive experience', WHO guideline on intrapartum care, 15 February 2018. https://www.who.int/reproductivehealth/intrapartum-care/en/

2    'Beyond too little, too late and too much, too soon: a pathway towards evidence-based, respectful maternity care worldwide', Suellen Miller et al., *The Lancet*, vol. 388, 29 October 2018. https://www.thelancet.com/journals/lancet/article/PIIS0140-6736(16)31472-6/fulltext

## CHAPTER 1

1    As quoted in *The Best Liberal Quotes Ever : Why the Left is Right*, William P. Martin, Sourcebooks, Chicago 2004

2    Survey conducted by the charity 4children in 2011, as reported on the NHS website. https://www.nhs.uk/news/pregnancy-and-child/postnatal-depression-often-unreported/

3    Research carried out by academics at City, University of London, in 2017. https://www.city.ac.uk/news/2017/february/maternal-ptsd-could-affect-up-to-28,000-women-in-the-uk-each-year,-says-new-review

4    *This is Going to Hurt*, Adam Kay, Picador, London 2018

5     https://www.dailymail.co.uk/health/article-6994943/Meghan-Markle-sparks-debate-global-obstetrics-summit.html

6    'Are middle-class "birthzillas" harassing hospital staff?', Kitty Holland, *Irish Times*, 4 May 2018. https://www.irishtimes.com/news/social-affairs/are-middle-class-birthzillas-harassing-hospital-staff-1.3484471

7    As published in an article on ethics.org.au in 2016. http://www.ethics.org.au/on-ethics/blog/august-2016/don%E2%80%99t-throw-the-birth-plan-out-with-the-bath-water

8    'The paradox of "safer" childbirth', Sheila Wayman, *Irish Times*, 26 June 2018. https://www.irishtimes.com/life-and-style/health-family/the-paradox-of-safer-childbirth-1.3535891

9    As quoted in a 2012 birthtalk.org online article. https://birthtrauma-truths.wordpress.com/2012/03/26/the-pitfalls-of-going-with-the-flow-in-birth/

10   Online survey carried out by Positive Birth Movement and Channel Mum in 2016. https://www.positivebirthmovement.org/birth-survey-2016/

11   'Bearing witness: United States and Canadian maternity support workers' observations of disrespectful care in childbirth', Christine H. Morton et al., *Birth Issues in Perinatal Care*, vol. 45, issue 3, 30 July 2018. https://onlinelibrary.wiley.com/doi/pdf/10.1111/birt.12373

12   'Doctor's comments on births at home angers group', *Irish Times*, 12 June 1996. https://www.irishtimes.com/news/doctor-s-comments-on-births-at-home-angers-group-1.57517

13   *Of Woman Born: Motherhood as Experience and Institution*, Adrienne Rich, W. W. Norton & Company, New York, 1976

14   '"Kidnapped" by the authorities: meet the woman forced to have a caesarean', Beverley Turner and Milli Hill, the *Telegraph*, 17 April 2014. https://www.telegraph.co.uk/women/mother-tongue/10767161/Kidnapped-by-the-authorities-meet-the-woman-forced-to-have-a-caesarean.html

15   https://www.globalhealthrights.org/wp-content/uploads/2013/03/EWCA-1997-Re-MB-Medical-Treatment.pdf

16    https://www.theguardian.com/world/2018/apr/15/caroline-criado-
      perez-suffragist-parliament-square-interview-millicent-fawcett-
      statue

17    'Development of self-control in children aged 3 to 9 years: Persp-
      ective from a dual-systems model', Ting Tao, Ligang Wang,
      Chunlei Fan and Wenbin Gao, published in *Nature* Scientific
      Reports vol. 4, Article no. 7272 (2014). https://www.nature.com/
      articles/srep07272

18    'The Bad News on "Good" Girls"', Jill Filipovic, *New York Times*
      November 2017. https://www.nytimes.com/2017/11/24/opinion/
      sunday/girls-parents-boys-gender.html

19    'Humanising Birth: Does the language we use matter?', Natalie
      Mobbs et al., *British Medical Journal* blog, 8 February 2018.
      https://blogs.bmj.com/bmj/2018/02/08/humanising-birth-does-
      the-language-we-use-matter/

20    'D-WORD ROW Midwives BANNED from saying "good girl" and
      "delivered" because they are disrespectful to pregnant woman',
      Jon Rogers, *Sun*, 9 February 2018. https://www.thesun.co.uk/
      news/5542921/midwives-banned-from-saying-good-girl-and-
      delivered-because-they-are-disrespectful-to-pregnant-woman/

21    https://www.mumsnet.com/Talk/am_i_being_unreasona-
      ble/1561173-To-hate-it-when-midwives-say-good-girl-when-
      women-are-giving-birth

22    'Cruelty in Maternity Wards: Fifty Years Later', *Journal of Perinatal
      Education*, 2010 summer, 19(3): 33–42. https://www.ncbi.nlm.nih.
      gov/pmc/articles/PMC2920649/

23    As reported in 'Forced episiotomy: Kelly's story', *Transformation*,
      Hermine Hayes-Klein, 10 September 2014. https://www.open-
      democracy.net/transformation/hermine-hayesklein/forced-episi-
      otomy-kelly's-story

24    'Listening to mothers III: report of the third national U.S. survey of
      women's childbearing experiences'. http://transform.childbirth-
      connection.org/reports/listeningtomothers/

25    As translated in 'Moving beyond disrespect and abuse: addressing
      the structural dimensions of obstetric violence', M Sadler et al.

*Reproductive Health Matters* 2016; X. https://eubirthresearch.files. wordpress.com/2015/09/wg4-moving-beyond-disrespect-and-abuse.pdf

26    Ibid

27    *The Lancet* Maternal Health Series, Prof. Oona Campbell et al., 2016. http://www.maternalhealthseries.org/explore-the-series/too-lit-tle-too-late/

28    *The Lancet* Maternal Health Series, Prof. Oona Campbell et al., 2016. http://www.maternalhealthseries.org/explore-the-series/too-much-too-soon/

29    'Making childbirth a positive experience: New WHO guideline on intrapartum care', 15 February 2018. https://www.who.int/ reproductivehealth/intrapartum-care/en/

30    'A "good birth" goes beyond having a healthy baby', Dr Princess Nothemba Simelela, WHO Assistant Director-General for Family, Women, Children and Adolescents, WHO Commentary, 15 February 2018. https://www.who.int/mediacentre/commentar-ies/2018/having-a-healthy-baby/en/

31    'Cruelty in Maternity Wards: Fifty Years Later', *Journal of Perinatal Education*, 2010 summer, 19(3): 33–42. https://www.ncbi.nlm.nih. gov/pmc/articles/PMC2920649/

32    'Making Loud Bodies "Feminine": A Feminist-Phenomenological Analysis of Obstetric Violence', Sara Cohen Shabot, *Human Studies* 39(2), 2015. https://www.researchgate.net/publication/-283286083_Making_Loud_Bodies_Feminine_A_Feminist-Phe-nomenological_Analysis_of_Obstetric_Violence

33    'Domesticating Bodies: The Role of Shame in Obstetric Violence', Sara Cohen Shabot and Keshet Korem, *Hypatia* vol. 33(3) summer 2018. https://onlinelibrary.wiley.com/doi/abs/10.1111/ hypa.12428

34    'Who owns the baby? A video ethnography of skin-to-skin contact after a caesarean section', Jeni Stevens et al., *Women and Birth* vol. 31, Issue 6, December 2018. https://www.sciencedirect.com/ science/article/pii/S1871519217302408?dgcid=coauthor

35    https://www.positivebirthmovement.org/about/our-campaigns/

36   *This is Going to Hurt*, Adam Kay, Picador, London 2018

37   'The First Hour Following Birth: Don't Wake the Mother!',
     Michael Odent, *Midwifery Today*, Issue 61, Spring 2002.
     https://midwiferytoday.com/mt-articles/first-hour/

38   Ibid

39   'Procedure in the NICU Uppsala, University Hospital Sweden',
     https://www.youtube.com/watch?v=VVwbVJpfgAc

40   'Mothers' Experiences of Initiating Lactation and Establishing
     Breastfeeding in a Neonatal Intensive Care Environment', C.
     Bartle, 2005. Unpublished Masters research thesis, University of
     Otago, New Zealand

41   'Victory Voyage: The Story of Evan', Natalie Dybisz, Positive Birth
     Movement.org. https://www.positivebirthmovement.org/victory-
     voyage-the-story-of-evan/

42   http://www.birthrights.org.uk/wordpress/wp-content/
     uploads/2018/08/Final-Birthrights-MRCS-Report-2108.pdf

43   'Why do women request an elective cesarean delivery for non-med-
     ical reasons? A systematic review of the qualitative literature',
     Charles O'Donovan and James O'Donovan, *Birth* vol. 45,
     November 2017. https://www.researchgate.net/publication/-
     320906460_Why_do_women_request_an_elective_cesar-
     ean_delivery_for_non-medical_reasons_A_systematic_review_
     of_the_qualitative_literature

44   'Let's tell the truth about caesareans – I had one and it was great',
     Natasha Pearlman, *The Sunday Times*, 23 August 2018. https://
     www.thetimes.co.uk/article/my-caesarean-was-great-i-
     want-other-women-to-have-that-choice-9h777sxm3

45   http://www.mamabirdbaby.com/blog/2018/7/28/freebirth-is-
     a-feminist-statement-mama-bird-doula

46   As reported in 'Why do some women choose to freebirth? A
     meta-thematic synthesis, part one', Claire Feeley et al.,
     *Evidence Based Midwifery*, 2015. https://www.rcm.org.uk/
     learning-and-career/learning-and-research/ebm-articles/why-
     do-some-women-choose-to-freebirth

47    'Why do some women choose to freebirth in the UK? An inter-
      pretative phenomenological study', Feeley and Thomson, *BMC
      Pregnancy and Childbirth*, 2016. https://bmcpregnancychildbirth.
      biomedcentral.com/articles/10.1186/s12884-016-0847-6

## CHAPTER 2

1    *The Whole Woman*, Germaine Greer, Doubleday, New York, 1999

2    *The Female Eunuch*, Germaine Greer, MacGibbon & Kee Ltd, London,
     1970.

3    As quoted in *The Whole Woman*, Germaine Greer, Doubleday, New
     York, 1999

4    *Of Woman Born: Motherhood as Experience and Institution*, Adrienne
     Rich, W.W. Norton & Company, New York and London, 1976

5    *How to Be a Woman*, Caitlin Moran, Ebury Press, London 2011

6    'Everything you wanted to know about fourth wave feminism–but
     were afraid to ask', Jessica Abrahams, *Prospect*, 14 August 2017
     https://www.prospectmagazine.co.uk/magazine/everything-
     wanted-know-fourth-wave-feminism

7    *Misconceptions: Truth, Lies, and the Unexpected on the Journey to
     Motherhood*, Naomi Wolf, Doubleday, New York, 2001

8    'To Reduce C-Sections, Change the Culture of the Labor Ward', Amy
     Dockser Marcus, The *Wall Street Journal*, 12 September 2017
     https://www.wsj.com/articles/to-reduce-c-sections-change-the-
     culture-of-the-labor-ward-1505268661

9    'How I added my voice to the war cry of millions of women who have
     given birth before me', Clementine Ford, *Sydney Morning Herald*,
     31 August 2016

10   'The fourth wave of feminism: meet the rebel women', Kira Cochrane,
     *Guardian*, 10 December 2013. https://www.theguardian.com/
     world/2013/dec/10/fourth-wave-feminism-rebel-women

11   *The Second Sex*, Simone de Beauvoir, first published in French in
     1949, Editions Gallimard, Paris. Second English translation by
     Constance Borde and Sheila Malovany-Chevallier, Knopf, New
     York, 2009

12    'Laurie Penny: "Women shouldn't apologise for the pitter-patter of tiny carbon footprints"', Laurie Penny, *Guardian*, 28 July 2017. https://www.theguardian.com/books/2017/jul/28/laurie-penny-women-shouldnt-apologise-for-carbon-footprints

13    Interview with Lisa Allardice, *Guardian*, 28 April 2018. https://www.theguardian.com/books/2018/apr/28/chimamanda-ngozi-adichie-feminism-racism-sexism-gender-metoo

14    'The obsession with "natural" birth is just another way to judge a woman', Hadley Freeman, *Guardian*, 29 May 2015 https://www.theguardian.com/commentisfree/2015/may/29/obsession-natural-birth-judge-women-pregnant-medical

15    'The cult of natural childbirth has gone too far', Eliane Glaser, *Guardian*, 5 March 2015. https://www.theguardian.com/commentisfree/2015/mar/05/natural-childbirth-report-midwife-musketeers-morcambe-bay

16    'Student athlete hazing victims may number 800,000 per year', Jessica Glenza, *Guardian*, 13 October 2014. https://www.theguardian.com/sport/2014/oct/13/student-athlete-hazing-victims-800000-per-year

17    'Natural childbirth ideology is endangering women and babies', Hans Peter Dietz, Lynda Exton, *Obstetrics & Gynecology*, vol.56, issue 5, October 2016. https://obgyn.onlinelibrary.wiley.com/doi/abs/10.1111/ajo.12524

18    'My NCT classes were so concerned with pushing an agenda they forgot to mention the realities of childbirth', Shannon Kyle, *Independent*, 19 April 2016. https://www.independent.co.uk/voices/my-nct-classes-were-so-concerned-with-pushing-an-agenda-they-forgot-to-mention-the-realities-of-a6991321.html

19    https://www.npeu.ox.ac.uk/mbrrace-uk/reports

20    '#Metoo shows we need trauma-informed maternity care', Rebecca Schiller, birthrights.org.uk, 20 October 2017. http://www.birthrights.org.uk/2017/10/metoo-shows-we-need-trauma-informed-maternity-care/

21    *The Guilty Feminist podcast*, episode 117 'Taking control of the narrative', Deborah Frances-White

22    'Childbirth stories are the stuff of life. We should share them', Eva Wiseman, *Guardian*, 8 April 2018. https://www.theguardian.com/lifeandstyle/2018/apr/08/lets-give-our-childbirth-stories-a-big-push-share-eve-wiseman

23    '"I felt I was being punished for pushing back": pregnancy and #MeToo', Justine van der Leun, *Guardian*, 17 March 2017. https://www.theguardian.com/lifeandstyle/2018/mar/17/punished-pushing-back-pregnancy-metoo

24    'From Metaphor to Legal Idiom: The Depiction of Women as "Vessels" in Antiquity and its Implications for 4Q416', David Rothstein, *Journal for Ancient Near Eastern and Biblical Law*, vol.13, 2007. https://www.jstor.org/stable/10.13173/zeitalto-biblrech.13.2007.0056?

25    'Forced C-section was "the stuff of nightmares": Social Services condemned for forcibly removing unborn child from woman', Chloe Hamilton, *Independent*, 1 December 2013. https://www.independent.co.uk/news/uk/home-news/social-services-forcibly-remove-unborn-child-from-woman-by-caesarean-after-she-suffered-mental-8975808.html

26    'Timeline of Savita Halappanavar's treatment: AIMS Ireland', *Assosiation for Improvements in the Maternity Services – Ireland*. http://aimsireland.ie/timeline-of-savita-halappanavars-treatment-aims-ireland/

27    As reported in '"You can do anything": Trump brags on tape about using fame to get women', Ben Jacobs, Sabrina Siddiqui, Scott Bixby, *Guardian*, 8 October 2016. https://www.theguardian.com/us-news/2016/oct/07/donald-trump-leaked-recording-women

28    As reported on the BBC news website, 2 October 2018. https://www.bbc.co.uk/news/av/world-us-canada-45712545/brett-kavanaugh-very-scary-time-for-young-men-in-america-trump

# CHAPTER 3

1   *Immaculate Deception: A New Look at Women and Childbirth in America*, Suzanne Arms, Houghton Mifflin, Boston, 1975

2   'What matters to women during childbirth: A systematic qualitative review', Soo Downe et al., *PLOS ONE*, 17 April 2018 https://journals.plos.org/plosone/article?id=10.1371/journal.pone.0194906

3   *Women and Power: A Manifesto*, Mary Beard, Profile Books, London, 2017

4   'Beyond too little, too late and too much, too soon: a pathway towards evidence-based, respectful maternity care worldwide', Suellen Miller et al., *The Lancet*, vol.388, issue 10056, 29 October 2016. https://www.thelancet.com/pdfs/journals/lancet/PIIS0140-6736(16)31472-6.pdf

5   As published in 'Optimising caesarean section use', *The Lancet*, 12 October 2018. https://www.thelancet.com/series/caesarean-section

6   'Proportion of induced labours rise', Julie Griffiths, rcm.org.uk, 26 October 2018. https://www.rcm.org.uk/news-views-and-analysis/news/proportion-of-induced-labours-rise

7   New European Perinatal Health Report released by the Euro-Peristat project, November 2018. https://www.europeristat.com/images/2018_11_26_PR_PerinatHealthFrEU2015_V2.pdf

8   *Interventions in Normal Labour and Birth*, RCM survey report March 2016. https://www.rcm.org.uk/sites/default/files/Labour%20Interventions%20Report.pdf

9   'Motherhood Is Hard to Get Wrong. So Why Do So Many Moms Feel So Bad About Themselves?', Claire Howorth, *Time*, 19 October 2017. http://time.com/4989068/motherhood-is-hard-to-get-wrong/

10  *Witches, Midwives & Nurses: A History of Women Healers*, Barbara Ehrenreich and Deirdre English, the Feminist Press, New York, 1973

11  'Oklahoma lawmakers want men to approve all abortions', Jordan Smith, *The Intercept*, 13 February 2017. https://theintercept.

com/2017/02/13/oklahoma-lawmakers-want-men-to-approve-all-abortions/

12 'GOP Florida law maker apologises for calling a pregnant woman a "host"', Amy Russo, *Huffington Post*, 1 March 2019. https://www.huffingtonpost.co.uk/entry/jose-oliva-host-abortion_n_5c7962ffe4b0de0c3fc06257

13 *Of Woman Born: Motherhood as Experience and Institution*, Adrienne Rich, W.W. Norton & Company, New York and London, 1976.

14 http://www.thebusinessofbeingborn.com/

15 https://archive.org/details/treatiseonartofm00nihe/

16 Ibid

17 https://www.nhs.uk/conditions/epidural/side-effects/

18 'Intrapartum care for healthy women and babies', NICE Clinical guideline 190, December 2014, updated February 2017. https://www.nice.org.uk/guidance/cg190/ifp/chapter/pain-relief

19 'Hormones in labour: Oxytocin, prolactin and what they are really doing', nct.org.uk, https://www.nct.org.uk/labour-birth/your-guide-labour/hormones-labour

20 'Pain management for women in labour – an overview of systematic reviews', L. Jones et al., Cochrane Database of Systematic Reviews 2012, Issue 3. https://www.cochrane.org/CD009234/PREG_pain-management-for-women-in-labour

21 'The effect of intrapartum pethidine on breastfeeding: a scoping review', Tanya Burchell et al., rcm.org.uk, 30 June 2016. https://www.rcm.org.uk/learning-and-career/learning-and-research/ebm-articles/the-effect-of-intrapartum-pethidine-on

22 'Choice of instruments for assisted vaginal delivery', F. O'Mahony et al., Cochrane Database of Systematic Reviews 2010, Issue 11. https://www.cochrane.org/CD005455/PREG_instruments-for-assisted-vaginal-delivery

23 'Epidural versus non-epidural or no analgesia for pain management in labour', M. Anim-Somuah et al., Cochrane Database of Systematic Reviews 2018, Issue 5. https://www.cochrane.org/CD000331/PREG_epidurals-pain-relief-labour

24  *Ina May's Guide to Childbirth*, Ina May Gaskin, Random House, New York, 2003

25  'Main determinants of maternal satisfaction after epidural analgesia for labour', A. Camaiora Kollman et al., *European Journal of Anaesthesiology*, June 2013 vol. 30. https://journals.lww.com/ejanaesthesiology/Fulltext/2013/06001/Main_determinants_of_maternal_satisfaction_after.529.aspx

26  'Investigating determinants for patient satisfaction in women receiving epidural analgesia for labour pain: a retrospective cohort study', Daryl Jian An Tan et al., *BMC Anesthesiology*, vol. 18, May 2018. https://www.ncbi.nlm.nih.gov/pmc/articles/PMC5944055/

27  'Epidurals – Dead from the waist down', Beverley A. Lawrence Beech, *AIMS Journal* 1998, vol. 10, no.1. https://www.aims.org.uk/journal/item/epidurals-dead-from-the-waist-down

28  https://www.youtube.com/watch?v=rlj9ehB-hLc

29  'Continuous support for women during childbirth', M.A. Bohren et al., Cochrane Database of Systematic Reviews 2017, Issue 7. https://www.cochrane.org/CD003766/PREG_continuous-support-women-during-childbirth

30  'Relationships: the pathway to safe, high-quality maternity care', J. Sandall et al. (writing on behalf of the Sheila Kitzinger symposium), report from the Sheila Kitzinger symposium at Green Templeton College, Oxford, October 2015. https://www.gtc.ox.ac.uk/wp-content/uploads/2018/12/skp_report.pdf

31  *The Politics of the Body: Gender in a Neoliberal and Neoconservative Age*, Alison Phipps, Polity Press, Cambridge, 2014

32  'Motherhood Is Hard to Get Wrong. So Why Do So Many Moms Feel So Bad About Themselves?', Claire Howorth, *Time*, 19 October 2017. http://time.com/4989068/motherhood-is-hard-to-get-wrong/

33  *The Angel in the House*, Coventry Patmore, John W. Parker and Son, London, 1858

34    'Professions for Women', Virginia Woolf, 1931, available in *The Death of the Moth, and Other Essays*, Harcourt Publishers Ltd, San Diego, 1974

35    'British maternal mortality in the 19 and early 20 centuries', Geoffrey Chamberlain, *Journal of the Royal Society of Medicine*, November 2006. https://www.ncbi.nlm.nih.gov/pmc/articles/PMC1633559/

36    https://www.atlasobscura.com/articles/twilight-sleep-child-birth-1910s-feminists

37    *Childbirth Without Fear*, Grantly Dick-Read, Heinemann Medical Books, 1942. Second edition, Pinter & Martin Ltd, London, 2013

38    As quoted in 'Prunella Briance obituary', Joanna Moorhead, *Guardian*, 22 August 2017. https://www.theguardian.com/life-andstyle/2017/aug/22/prunella-briance-obituary

39    Cited in *The Experience of Childbirth*, Sheila Kitzinger, Victor Gollancz, London, 1962. Second edition, *The New Experience of Childbirth*, Orion, London, 2004

40    'Prunella Briance obituary', Joanna Moorhead, *Guardian*, 22 August 2017. https://www.theguardian.com/lifeandstyle/2017/aug/22/prunella-briance-obituary

41    *The Experience of Childbirth*, Sheila Kitzinger, Victor Gollancz, London, 1962. Second edition, *The New Experience of Childbirth*, Orion, London, 2004

42    http://thefarmmidwives.org/

43    Updated statistics on The Farm website: http://thefarmmidwives.org/preliminary-statistics/
Background USA statistics from footnote were accessed here:
Home birth rate: https://www.acog.org/Clinical-Guidance-and-Publications/Committee-Opinions/Committee-on-Obstetric-Practice/Planned-Home-Birth?
Caesarean rate: https://www.cdc.gov/nchs/fastats/delivery.htm
Neonatal mortality: https://www.healthsystemtracker.org/chart-collection/infant-mortality-u-s-compare-coun-tries/#item-infant-mortality-higher-u-s-comparable-countries
Maternal mortality concern: https://www.nationalgeographic.

com/culture/2018/12/maternal-mortality-usa-health-mother
hood/

44 'Active Management of Labour', Kieran O'Driscoll et al., *British Medical Journal*, 1973 vol. 3. https://www.ncbi.nlm.nih.gov/pmc/articles/PMC1586344/pdf/brmedj01567-0029.pdf

45 https://midwifethinking.com/2015/05/02/vaginal-examinations-a-symptom-of-a-cervix-centric-birth-culture

46 https://www.maternityworldwide.org/what-we-do/three-delays-model/

47 'Choice, policy and practice in maternity care since 1948', history-andpolicy.org, Angela Davis, 30 May 2013. http://www.history-andpolicy.org/policy-papers/papers/choice-policy-and-practice-in-maternity-care-since-1948

48 'Proportion of induced labours rise', Julie Griffiths, rcm.org.uk, 26 October 2018. https://www.rcm.org.uk/news-views-and-analysis/news/proportion-of-induced-labours-rise

49 'Episiotomy during childbirth: not just a "little snip"', *The Conversation*, 15 January, 2015. https://theconversation.com/episiotomy-during-childbirth-not-just-a-little-snip-36062

50 'Retrospective analysis of episiotomy prevalence', Bahtışen Kartal et al., *Journal of the Turkish-German Gynecological Association*, December 2017. https://www.ncbi.nlm.nih.gov/pmc/articles/PMC5776158/

51 'The Husband Stitch', Carmen Maria Machado, *Granta* 129: Fate, 28 October 2014. https://granta.com/the-husband-stitch/

52 'Episiotomies Still Common During Childbirth Despite Advice To Do Fewer', Jocelyn Wiener, npr.org, 4 July 2016. https://www.npr.org/sections/health-shots/2016/07/04/483945168/episiotomies-still-common-during-childbirth-despite-advice-to-do-fewer?t=1540375207264

53 'The "Husband Stitch" Leaves Women in Pain and Without Answers', Mary Halton, *Broadly*, 26 April 2018. https://broadly.vice.com/en_us/article/pax95m/the-husband-stitch-real-stories-episiotomy

54 'The Husband Stitch Isn't Just a Horrifying Childbirth Myth', Carrie Murphy, *Healthline*, 24 January 2018. https://www.healthline. com/health-news/husband-stitch-is-not-just-myth#1

55 http://www.roda.hr/en/reports/complaints-sent-to-un-bodies-on-obstetric-violence-in-croatia

56 'The Evolution of Maternal Birthing Position', Lauren Dundes, *American Journal of Public Health*, May 1987, vol. 77, no. 5. https://ajph.aphapublications.org/doi/pdf/10.2105/AJPH.77.5.636

57 'The bizarre reason why women started giving birth lying down', Mahalia Chang, *Now to Love*, 28 February 2018. https://www. nowtolove.com.au/parenting/pregnancy-birth/lying-down-birth-history-45385

58 'The Evidence on: Birthing Positions', Rebecca Dekker, evidence-basedbirth.com, October 2012, updated 2 February 2018. https://evidencebasedbirth.com/evidence-birthing-positions/

59 https://www.cqc.org.uk/publications/surveys/maternity-services-survey-2018

60 'The Evidence on: Birthing Positions', Rebecca Dekker, evidence-basedbirth.com, October 2012, updated 2 February 2018. https://evidencebasedbirth.com/evidence-birthing-positions/

61 'Stand and deliver – upright births best for mum and bub', Hannah Dahlen, *The Conversation*, 6 May 2013. https://theconversation. com/stand-and-deliver-upright-births-best-for-mum-and-bub-13095

62 'Janet Balaskas: campaigner for active birth movement', Claire Bowes, BBC World Service, 4 April 2012. https://www.bbc.co.uk/news/health-17589544

63 https://www.cqc.org.uk/publications/surveys/maternity-services-survey-2018

64 Data from CDC report quoted in 'How Many Women Are Getting Epidurals Now Compared To Previous Generations? The Majority Do', Mara Flanagan, Romper.com, 30 September 2016. https://www.romper.com/p/how-many-women-are-getting-epidurals-now-compared-to-previous-generations-the-majority-do-19464

65 'Why do so many French women have epidurals?', *The Local*, 1 September 2015. https://www.thelocal.fr/20150904/why-do-so-many-french-women-have-epidurals

66 'The Effect of Epidural Analgesia on the Delivery Outcome of Induced Labour: A Retrospective Case Series', Angeliki Antonakou and Dimitrios Papoutsis, *Obstetrics and Gynecology International*, November, 2016. https://www.ncbi.nlm.nih.gov/pmc/articles/PMC5136389/

67 'Epidural versus non-epidural or no analgesia for pain management in labour', M. Anim-Somuah et al., Cochrane Database of Systematic Reviews May 2018, Issue 5. https://www.cochrane.org/CD000331/PREG_epidurals-pain-relief-labour

68 'Get the Epidural', Jessi Klein, *The New York Times*, 9 July 2016. https://www.nytimes.com/2016/07/10/opinion/sunday/get-the-epidural.html

69 *Of Woman Born: Motherhood as Experience and Institution*, Adrienne Rich, W.W. Norton & Company, New York and London, 1976

70 'Indemnity provision for IMUK midwives is "inappropriate", says NMC', nmc.org.uk, 13 January 2017. https://www.nmc.org.uk/news/news-and-updates/indemnity-provision-for-imuk-midwives-is-inappropriate-says-nmc/

71 *Rediscovering Birth*, Sheila Kitzinger, Little, Brown, London, 2000. Revised edition Pinter & Martin, London, 2011

72 As discussed in *Childbirth and Authoritative Knowledge: Cross Cultural Perspectives*, Robbie E. Davis-Floyd, University of California Press, California, 1997

73 'Intuition as Authoritative Knowledge in Midwifery and Homebirth', Robbie Davis-Floyd, *Medical Anthropology Quarterly*, June 1996. https://www.researchgate.net/profile/Robbie_Davis-Floyd/publication/227668442_Intuition_as_Authoritative_Knowledge_in_Midwifery_and_Homebirth/links/0fcfd511ea267c4902000000.pdf

74 'Emotion work in midwifery: a review of current knowledge', Billie Hunter, *Journal of Advanced Nursing*, vol. 34, issue 4, May 2001. https://onlinelibrary.wiley.com/doi/abs/10.1046/j.1365-2648.2001.01772.x

75 'Getting To Grips With The "Normal" Birth Debate', Soo Downe, *Huffpost*, 19 October 2017. https://www.huffingtonpost.co.uk/soo-downe-obe/getting-to-grips-with-the_1_b_18227714.html

76 'Midwife-led continuity models versus other models of care for childbearing women', J. Sandall et al., Cochrane Database of Systematic Reviews, 2016, Issue 4. https://www.cochrane.org/CD004667/PREG_midwife-led-continuity-models-care-compared-other-models-care-women-during-pregnancy-birth-and-early

77 'Relationships: the pathway to safe, high-quality maternity care', J. Sandall et al (writing on behalf of the Sheila Kitzinger symposium), report from the Sheila Kitzinger symposium at Green Templeton College, Oxford, October 2015. https://www.gtc.ox.ac.uk/wp-content/uploads/2018/12/skp_report.pdf

78 https://www.england.nhs.uk/wp-content/uploads/2016/02/national-maternity-review-report.pdf

79 As reported in 'U.S. "Most Dangerous" Place To Give Birth In Developed World, USA Today Investigation Finds', CBS Chicago, 26 July 2018. https://chicago.cbslocal.com/2018/07/26/u-s-most-dangerous-place-give-birth/

80 'Doctor claims midwives are putting babies' lives at risk with their alternative methods and "dark arts"', Andrew Prentice, *Daily Mail Australia*, 17 August 2018. https://www.dailymail.co.uk/news/article-6069237/Adelaide-doctor-questions-controversial-courses-midwives-assist-child-birth.html

81 https://ama.com.au/media/obstetricians-and-gp-obstetricians-excluded-maternity-care-disturbing-trend-ama-0?

82 https://ama.com.au/media/maternity-services-must-be-obstetric-led?

83 https://www.facebook.com/maternityconsumernetwork/posts/789473558059431?

# CHAPTER 4

1   *Burning Woman*, Lucy H. Pearce, Womancraft Publishing, Cork, 2016

2   www.positivebirthmovement.org

3   'Ethics of the delivery room: Who's in control when you're giving birth?', Rebecca Grant, *Independent*, 18 December 2017. https://www.independent.co.uk/news/long_reads/childbirth-delivery-room-ethics-doctor-patient-healthcare-a8085346.html

4   'Interview: The women hounded for giving birth outside the system', Rebecca Schiller, *Guardian*, 22 October 2016. https://www.theguardian.com/lifeandstyle/2016/oct/22/hounded-for-giving-birth-outside-the-system

5   'A Happy Ending for Free Birth Mother Thanks to Concerned "Trolls"', Katie Joy, *Without a Crystal Ball*, 30 October 2018. https://www.patheos.com/blogs/withoutacrystal-ball/2018/10/14652/

6   'She Wanted a "Freebirth" at Home. When the Baby Died, the Attacks Began', Emily Shugerman, *Daily Beast*, 11 March 2018. https://www.thedailybeast.com/she-wanted-a-freebirth-at-home-when-the-baby-died-the-attacks-began

7   https://www.tv3.lt/naujiena/lietuva/973469/nekasdiene-istorija-gim-dymo-namuose-moters-elgesys-nustebino-visko-maciusius?

8   https://www.15min.lt/naujiena/aktualu/nusikaltimaiirnelaimes/siauliu-patruliai-iskviesti-i-gimdyma-medikai-nesusit-varke-su-emocinga-gimdyve-59-1026226?

9   '"You did not cry when you had sex, so shut up": Balkan women share agonising #MeToo gynaecology stories', *Telegraph*, 2 January 2019. https://www.telegraph.co.uk/news/2019/01/02/did-not-cry-had-sex-shut-balkan-women-share-agonising-metoo/

10  'Violent Treatment During Childbirth: Croatian Women Speak Out', Anja Vladisavljevic, *Balkan Insight*, 1 November 2018. https://balkaninsight.com/2018/11/01/violent-treatment-during-child-birth-croatian-women-speak-out-10-31-2018/?

11  'York – it's not for women', Emma Ashworth, *AIMS Journal*, vol. 30, no. 3, 2018. https://www.aims.org.uk/journal/item/york-home-birth

12  *The Handmaid's Tale*, Margaret Atwood, McClelland and Stewart, Toronto, 1985

13  https://imuk.org.uk/

14  'Outcomes for births booked under an independent midwife and births in NHS maternity units: matched comparison study', Andrew Symon et al., *British Medical Journal* 2009; 338:b2060. https://www.bmj.com/content/338/bmj.b2060

15  http://www.health.gov.au/internet/main/publishing.nsf/Content/midwives-nurse-pract-collaborative-arrangements

16  'Gaye Demanuele and the Politics of Homebirth', Petra Bueskens, *New Matilda*, 10 June 2016. https://newmatilda.com/2016/06/10/gaye-demanuele-and-the-politics-of-homebirth/

17  http://www.onetoonemidwives.org/

18  http://thealbanymodel.com/

19  https://www.midwifery.org.uk/news/maternity-care/albany-mid-wives-exonerated-arm-demands-apology/

20  'Perineal tearing is a national issue we must address', David Richmond, 11 July 2014, RDOG.org.uk. https://www.rcog.org.uk/en/blog/perineal-tearing-is-a-national-issue-we-must-address/

21  'Reclaiming birth rally', Nadine Edwards, *AIMS Journal*, vol. 22, no. 1, 2010. https://www.aims.org.uk/journal/item/reclaiming-birth-rally

22  'Midwifery continuity of carer in an area of high socio-economic disadvantage in London: A retrospective analysis of Albany Midwifery Practice outcomes using routine data (1997–2009)', Caroline S. E. Homer et al., *Midwifery*, vol. 48, May 2017. https://www.sciencedirect.com/science/article/pii/S0266613817301511#t0015

23  http://moderngov.southwark.gov.uk/mgConvert2PDF.aspx-?ID=10844

24  'Midwife is cleared after three-year "witch hunt"', Martin Barrow, *The Times*, 3 July 2013. https://www.thetimes.co.uk/article/midwife-is-cleared-after-three-year-witch-hunt-gc6xp0r95fs

25    'Agnes Gereb – yet another travesty', Lesley Page, all4maternity.com,
      1 February 2018. https://www.all4maternity.com/agnes-gereb-
      yet-another-travesty/

26    'President János Áder Pardons Homebirth Midwife Ágnes Geréb',
      Gábor Sarnyai, *Hungary Today*, 29 June 2018. https://hungaryto-
      day.hu/president-janos-ader-pardons-homebirth-midwife-agnes-
      gereb/

27    'European court decision boosts Gereb campaign_2', Gareth Price,
      rcm.org.uk, 15 December 2010. https://www.rcm.org.uk/news-
      views-and-analysis/news/european-court-decision-boosts-ger-
      eb-campaign2

28    'Midwife: "My 10 year fight to prove that cutting the cord too soon
      puts babies at risk"', Radhika Sanghani, *Telegraph*, 22 April 2015.
      https://www.telegraph.co.uk/health-fitness/body/midwife-my-
      10-year-fight-to-prove-that-cutting-the-cord-too-soon-puts-ba-
      bies-at-risk/

29    https://www.internationalmidwives.org/our-work/policy-and-prac-
      tice/icm-definitions.html

30    'Midwives to end campaign to promote "normal births"', George
      Sandeman, *Guardian*, 12 August 2017. https://www.theguardian.
      com/society/2017/aug/12/midwives-to-stop-using-term-normal-
      birth

31    'The Report of the Morecambe Bay Investigation', Dr Bill Kirkup
      CBE. https://assets.publishing.service.gov.uk/government/
      uploads/system/uploads/attachment_data/file/408480/47487_
      MBI_Accessible_v0.1.pdf

32    'Why UK midwives stopped the campaign for "normal birth"',
      Vanora Hundley and Edwin van Teijlingen, *The Conversation*,
      31 August 2017. https://theconversation.com/why-uk-midwives-
      stopped-the-campaign-for-normal-birth-82779

33    http://www.sheenabyrom.com/blog/2017/8/16/normal-birth-evi-
      dence-and-facts

34    'NHS trusts are STILL promoting natural births to mothers despite
      series of baby deaths being linked to the delivery method', Tom
      Witherow, *Daily Mail*, 20 November 2017. https://www.dailymail.

co.uk/health/article-5098885/NHS-trusts-promoting-natural-births.html

35   'Top midwife: Doctors "hopeless at childbirth"', Sarah-Kate Templeton, *Sunday Times*, 18 March 2018. https://www.thetimes.co.uk/article/top-midwife-doctors-hopeless-at-childbirth-b0kj809l0

36   'Women Describe Their Orgasmic Births', Rebecca Schiller, *Broadly*, 30 May 2016. https://broadly.vice.com/en_us/article/qkggd7/women-describe-their-orgasmic-births

37   *Birth and Sex: the power and the passion*, Sheila Kitzinger, Pinter & Martin Ltd, London, 2012

38   https://www.thesun.co.uk/fabulous/7679382/labour-mp-jess-phillips-girls-taught-orgasms-sex-education/

39   https://www.theguardian.com/commentisfree/2016/sep/15/3d-model-clitoris-sexual-revolution-sex-education-womens-sexuality

40   As reported in 'Megyn Kelly claims Donald Trump feud has "not been enjoyable" as she hints at leaving Fox News', Olivia Blair, *Independent*, 7 April 2016. https://www.independent.co.uk/news/people/megyn-kelly-wishes-donald-trump-would-stop-his-focus-on-me-as-she-hints-at-leaving-fox-news-a6972571.html

41   'Male appropriation and medicalization of childbirth: an historical analysis', H. A. Cahill, *Journal of Advanced Nursing*, vol. 33, no. 3, February 2001. https://www.ncbi.nlm.nih.gov/pubmed/11251720

## CHAPTER 5

1   *The Second Sex*, Simone de Beauvoir, first published in French in 1949, Editions Gallimard, Paris. Second English translation by Constance Borde and Sheila Malovany-Chevallier, Knopf, New York, 2009

2   'Worldwide prevalence of tocophobia in pregnant women: systematic review and meta-analysis', M. A. O'Connell et al., *Acta Obstetricia et Gynecologica Scandinavica*, vol. 96 no. 8, August 2017. https://www.ncbi.nlm.nih.gov/pubmed/28369672

3   'Survey of obstetricians' personal preference and discretionary practice', R. Al-Mufti et al., *European Journal of Obstetrics, Gyne-*

*cology and Reproductive Biology*, vol. 73, no. 1, May 1997. littpc://
www.ncbi.nlm.nih.gov/pubmed/9175681

4   'We know the reality of childbirth', Bridget O'Donnell, *Guardian*, 11
    July 2008. https://www.theguardian.com/society/2008/jul/11/nhs.
    health1

5   'Trauma and fear in Australian midwives', J. Toohill, et al., *Women
    Birth*, vol. 32, no. 1, February 2019. https://www.ncbi.nlm.nih.
    gov/m/pubmed/29759933/

6   'A Wider Pelvis Does Not Increase Locomotor Cost in Humans, with
    Implications for the Evolution of Childbirth', Anna G. Warrener
    et al., *PLoS ONE*, vol. 10, no. 3, 11 March 2015. https://journals.
    plos.org/plosone/article?id=10.1371/journal.pone.0118903

7   'There Is No "Obstetrical Dilemma": Towards a Braver Medicine with
    Fewer Childbirth Interventions', H. M. Dunsworth, *Perspectives
    in Biology and Medicine*, vol. 61, no. 2, 2018. https://www.ncbi.
    nlm.nih.gov/pubmed/30146522

8   'Metabolic hypothesis for human altriciality', Holly M. Dunsworth et
    al., *Proceedings of the National Academy of Sciences*, August 2012.
    https://www.pnas.org/content/early/2012/08/28/1205282109

9   'Difficult Labor: Birth Canal Issues', Rachel Nall, Healthline.com, 24
    February 2016. https://www.healthline.com/health/pregnancy/
    labor-birth-canal#treatment

10  'Cliff-edge model of obstetric selection', Philipp Mitteroecker et al.,
    *Proceedings of the National Academy of Sciences*, December 2016.
    https://www.pnas.org/content/113/51/14680

11  https://www.rcog.org.uk/en/patients/patient-leaflets/about-rcog-
    guidelines-and-parallel-information-for-the-public/

12  'Labor Induction versus Expectant Management in Low-Risk Nullip-
    arous Women', William A. Grobman et al., *New England Journal
    of Medicine*, vol. 379, 9 August 2018. https://www.nejm.org/doi/
    full/10.1056/NEJMoa1800566

13  'Does ARRIVE set the stage for 39-week induction?', Judith M.
    Orvos, *Contemporary OB/GYN*, 14 August 2018. https://www.
    contemporaryobgyn.net/labor-induction/does-arrive-set-stage-
    39-week-induction

14    'The ARRIVE Trial has finally arrived – a midwife's summary', Hannah Dahlen, all4maternity.com, 9 August 2018. https://www. all4maternity.com/the-arrive-trial-has-finally-arrived-a-mid-wifes-summary/

15    'Parsing the ARRIVE Trial: Should First-Time Parents Be Routinely Induced at 39 Weeks?', Henci Goer, science&sensibility.org. https://www.scienceandsensibility.org/blog/parsing-the-arrive-trial-should-first-time-parents-be-routinely-induced-at-39-weeks

16    'WHO recommendations for induction of labour', WHO.int, 2011, updated 2018. https://www.who.int/reproductivehealth/publica-tions/maternal_perinatal_health/9789241501156/en/

17    'Rise in women having induced labours, NHS figures show', bbc. co.uk, 25 October 2018. https://www.bbc.co.uk/news/health-45978623

18    'Membrane sweeping for induction of labour', M. Boulvain et al., *Cochrane Database of Systematic Reviews*, 2005, Issue 1. https:// www.cochranelibrary.com/cdsr/doi/10.1002/14651858.CD000451. pub2/epdf/full

19    'The Evidence on: Due Dates', Rebecca Dekker, evidencebasedbirth. com, 15 April 2015. https://evidencebasedbirth.com/evidence-on-inducing-labor-for-going-past-your-due-date/

20    *Why Induction Matters*, Rachel Reed, Pinter & Martin Ltd, London, 2018

21    'How accurate are "due dates"?', Keith Moore, bbc.co.uk, 3 February 2015. https://www.bbc.co.uk/news/magazine-31046144

22    'Induction of labour for improving birth outcomes for women at or beyond term', P. Middleton et al., Cochrane Database of Systematic Reviews, 2018, Issue 5. https://www.cochrane. org/CD004945/PREG_induction-labour-women-normal-pregnancies-or-beyond-term

23    https://www.nice.org.uk/guidance/cg70/chapter/1-Guidance#infor-mation-and-decision-making

24    'Aging of the placenta', H. Fox, *Archives of Disease in Childhood – Fetal and Neonatal Edition* vol. 77, 1997. https://fn.bmj.com/

content/77/3/F171?fbclid=IwAR00OTThnAdsdpuHuSO1Q-
2FuqRI-Fy0Rij8gmloiVxWcfaWe5i6ccACvkOE

25   'Rise in women having induced labours "because of Britain's obesity
crisis and soaring numbers of older mothers", NHS figures show',
Stephen Matthews, *Daily Mail*, 26 October 2018. https://www.
dailymail.co.uk/health/article-6319373/Rise-women-having-in-
duced-labours-NHS-figures-show.html

26   'Synthetic oxytocin linked to postnatal depression', Melinda
Rollinson, kidspot.com.au, 18 October 2017. https://www.
kidspot.com.au/birth/labour/types-of-birth/synthetic-oxy-
tocin-linked-to-postnatal-depression/news-story/2cd4a3234b1e-
124506f2b7fa746f5371

27   'The effect of medical and operative birth interventions on child
health outcomes in the first 28 days and up to 5 years of age:
A linked data population-based cohort study', Lilian L. Peters
et al., *Birth*, vol. 45, 2018. https://onlinelibrary.wiley.com/doi/
pdf/10.1111/birt.12348

28   'Is it possible to safely prevent late preterm and early term births?',
Scott W. White and John P. Newnham, *Seminars in Fetal and
Neonatal Medicine*, vol. 24, issue 1, February 2019. https://www.
sciencedirect.com/science/article/pii/S1744165X18301252

29   'Pre-term births on demand: UWA Professor John Newnham', Belle
Taylor, *Perth Now*, 3 November 2018. https://www.perthnow.com.
au/news/health/pre-term-births-on-demand-uwa-professor-
john-newnham-ng-b881003240z

30   'How would Mary Poppins fare in labour? Practically perfect? Unlikely', L. Bolger et al., *Irish Medical Journal*, May
2018. http://imj.ie/how-would-mary-poppins-fare-in-labour-
practically-perfect-unlikely/

31   'The Birthplace cohort study: key findings', National Perinatal Epidemiology Unit, updated 1 February 2017. https://www.npeu.ox.ac.
uk/birthplace/results

32   https://www.nice.org.uk/guidance/cg190/chapter/Recommenda-
tions#place-of-birth

33    'Where to give birth, at home or in a hospital? Does it matter?', Peter Brocklehurst, UCL Lunch Hour Lectures, 29 January 2013. https://www.youtube.com/watch?v=MP0oQjXFPio

34    'Home births three times more risky than hospital, says study', Hayden Smith, *Metro*, 24 November 2011. https://metro.co.uk/2011/11/24/home-births-are-three-times-more-risky-than-hospital-births-says-study-232377/

35    'First-time mothers who opt for home birth face triple the risk of death or brain damage in child', Jenny Hope, *Daily Mail*, 25 November 2011. https://www.dailymail.co.uk/health/article-2065928/First-time-mothers-opt-home-birth-face-triple-risk-death-brain-damage-child.html

36    *Domiciliary Midwifery and Maternity Bed Needs: Report of the Standing Maternity and Midwifery Advisory Committee*, Central Health Services Council (sub-committee Chairman J. Peel), HMSO, London, 1970

37    http://holisticmidwifery.com.au/

38    'Perineal tearing is a national issue we must address', David Richmond, rcog.org.uk, 11 July 2014. https://www.rcog.org.uk/en/blog/perineal-tearing-is-a-national-issue-we-must-address/

39    'Third- and Fourth-degree Perineal Tears, Management (Green-top Guideline No. 29)', rcog.org.uk, 12 June 2015. https://www.rcog.org.uk/en/guidelines-research-services/guidelines/gtg29/

40    'Midwifery continuity of carer in an area of high socio-economic disadvantage in London: A retrospective analysis of Albany Midwifery Practice outcomes using routine data (1997–2009)', Caroline S. E. Homer et al., *Midwifery*, vol. 48, May 2017. https://www.sciencedirect.com/science/article/pii/S0266613817301511

41    http://thefarmmidwives.org/preliminary-statistics/

42    *Ina May's Guide to Childbirth*, Ina May Gaskin, Random House, New York, 2003

43    OASI care bundle Scaling Up Programme, rcog.org.uk. https://www.rcog.org.uk/en/guidelines-research-services/audit-quality-improvement/oasi-care-bundle/

44 'Perineal protection during spontaneous labour', Lars HØJ, YouTube, 18 February 2014. https://www.youtube.com/watch?v=X9_FP3f-G8XM&t=2s

45 https://www.rcog.org.uk/en/guidelines-research-services/audit-quality-improvement/oasi-care-bundle/oasi-faqs/#perrectumhow

46 'The Perineal "Bundle" and Midwifery', Rachel Reed, midwifethinking.com, 9 May 2018, updated December 2018. https://midwifethinking.com/2018/05/09/the-perineal-bundle-and-midwifery/

47 'Congratulations on your new baby', Jim Thornton, ripe-tomato.org, 11 December 2018. https://ripe-tomato.org/2018/12/11/congratulations-on-your-new-baby/

48 https://www.rcog.org.uk/en/guidelines-research-services/audit-quality-improvement/oasi-care-bundle/oasi-faqs/#perrectumwhy

49 'Maternal and perinatal outcomes by planned place of birth among women with low-risk pregnancies in high-income countries: A systematic review and meta-analysis', Vanessa L. Scarf et al., *Midwifery*, vol. 62, 2018. https://www.midwiferyjournal.com/article/S0266-6138(18)30097-4/pdf

50 'Perineal techniques during the second stage of labour for reducing perineal trauma', V. Aasheim et al., Cochrane Database of Systematic Reviews 2017, Issue 6. https://www.cochrane.org/CD006672/PREG_perineal-techniques-during-second-stage-labour-reducing-perineal-trauma

51 'Continuous cardiotocography (CTG) as a form of electronic fetal monitoring (EFM) for fetal assessment during labour', Z. Alfirevic et al., Cochrane Database of Systematic Reviews 2017, Issue 2. https://www.cochrane.org/CD006066/PREG_continuous-cardiotocography-ctg-form-electronic-fetal-monitoring-efm-fetal-assessment-during-labour

52 'Electronic Fetal Heart Rate Monitoring: The Future', Taran Khangura and Edwin Chandraharan, *Current Women's Health Reviews* 2013, issue 9. https://www.researchgate.net/publication/263610566_Electronic_Fetal_Heart_Rate_Monitoring_The_Future

53   'Cardiotocography versus intermittent auscultation of fetal heart on admission to labour ward for assessment of fetal wellbeing', D. Devane et al., Cochrane Database of Systematic Reviews 2017, Issue 1. https://www.cochrane.org/CD005122/PREG_comparing-electronic-monitoring-babys-heartbeat-womans-admission-labour-using-cardiotocography-ctg

54   'Immersion in Water During Labor and Delivery', American College of Obstetricians and Gynecologists, Committee Opinion no. 679, November 2016. https://www.acog.org/Clinical-Guidance-and-Publications/Committee-Opinions/Committee-on-Obstetric-Practice/Immersion-in-Water-During-Labor-and-Delivery?IsMobileSet=false

55   'Having a water birth and using a birth pool', Which? Birth Choice, which.co.uk. https://www.which.co.uk/birth-choice/coping-with-pain-in-labour/having-a-water-birth-and-using-a-birth-pool

56   'Water births have no proven benefit and could be dangerous: Study highlights risk of infection and breathing problems for babies', Fiona MacRea, *Daily Mail*, 19 March 2014. https://www.dailymail.co.uk/health/article-2584760/Water-births-no-proven-benefit-dangerous-study-highlights-risk-infection-breathing-problems-babies.html

57   'Experts warn against at-home water births after mum shares video of herself giving birth in tub', Mariana Cerqueira, goodtoknow.co.uk, 15 August 2018. https://www.goodtoknow.co.uk/family/experts-warn-against-at-home-waterbirths-mum-shares-video-birth-in-tub-432330

58   From his essay in *Water Birth Unplugged: Proceedings of the First International Water Birth Conference*, Beverley A. Lawrence Beech (ed.), Books for Midwives, 1996

59   'Evidence grows that normal childbirth takes longer than we thought', Aimee Cunningham, *Science News*, 16 January 2018. https://www.sciencenews.org/article/evidence-grows-normal-childbirth-takes-longer-we-thought?fbclid

60   https://www.who.int/reproductivehealth/topics/maternal_perinatal/intrapartum-care-infographics/en/

61    'Evidence on: Prolonged Second Stage of Labor', Rebecca Dekker, Evidencebasedbirth.com, 24 May 2017. https://evidencebased-birth.com/prolonged-second-stage-of-labor/

62    'Do Not Disturb: The Importance of Privacy in Labor', Judith A. Lothian, *Journal of Perinatal Education*, vol. 13, no. 3, summer 2004. https://www.ncbi.nlm.nih.gov/pmc/articles/PMC1595201/#citeref3

63    '"I knew I was in labour" – why are women being turned away from hospital during childbirth?', Emine Saner, *Guardian*, 15 January 2018. https://www.theguardian.com/lifeandstyle/2018/jan/15/i-knew-i-was-in-labour-why-are-women-being-turned-away-from-hospital-during-childbirth

## CHAPTER 6

1    'Throwing Like a Girl: A Phenomenology of Feminine Body Comportment Motility and Spatiality', Iris Marion Young, *Human Studies*, vol. 3, 1980.

2    'By removing photos of childbirth, Facebook is censoring powerful female images', Milli Hill, *Guardian*, 22 October 2014. https://www.theguardian.com/commentisfree/2014/oct/22/facebook-re-moving-childbirth-female-images

3    'Burnt Norton', *Four Quartets*, T.S. Eliot, Faber and Faber, London, 1941.

4    'Model receives rape and death threats for showing unshaved legs in an Adidas advert', Ellen Scott, *Metro*, 7 October 2017. https://metro.co.uk/2017/10/07/model-receives-rape-and-death-threats-for-showing-unshaved-legs-in-an-adidas-advert-6983379/

5    'The Photographs of Women's Bodies That Instagram Censored', Molly Gottschalk, artsy.net, 13 March 2017. https://www.artsy.net/article/artsy-editorial-photographs-womens-bodies-insta-gram-censored

6    'Harnett mom banned from Facebook over her child breastfeeding photo', Renee Chou, WRAL.com, 8 November 2018. https://www.wral.com/mother-outraged-after-facebook-bans-breastfeed-ing-photo-/17979895/

7    'Mum ordered to breastfeed behind curtain to avoid causing offence', Richard Hartley-Parkinson, *Metro*, 13 February 2019. https://metro.co.uk/2019/02/13/mum-ordered-breastfeed-behind-curtain-avoid-causing-offence-8606260/

8    'Mum, 38, told it's inappropriate to breastfeed twins at nursery', Tanveer Mann, *Metro*, 22 January 2019. https://metro.co.uk/2019/01/22/mum-38-told-inappropriate-breastfeed-twins-nursery-8373603/

9    *The Female Eunuch*, Germaine Greer, MacGibbon & Kee Ltd, London, 1970

10   'Making loud bodies "feminine": a feminist-phenomenological analysis of obstetric violence', Sara Cohen Shabot, academia.edu. http://www.academia.edu/19975105/Making_loud_bodies_feminine_a_feminist-phenomenological_analysis_of_obstetric_violence

11   'Why do women request an elective cesarean delivery for non-medical reasons? A systematic review of the qualitative literature', Charles and James O'Donovan, *Birth* 45, November 2017. https://www.researchgate.net/publication/320906460_Why_do_women_request_an_elective_cesarean_delivery_for_non-medical_reasons_A_systematic_review_of_the_qualitative_literature

12   'WHO recommendation against routine perineal/pubic shaving prior to giving vaginal birth', WHO recommendation, 1 September 2015. https://extranet.who.int/rhl/topics/preconception-pregnancy-childbirth-and-postpartum-care/who-recommendation-against-routine-perineal/pubic-shaving-prior-giving-vaginal-birth

13   'Uncensored birth: Instagram updates their policy around childbirth photos', Heather Marcoux, *Motherly*, 17 May 2018. https://www.mother.ly/news/uncensored-birth-instagram-updates-policy-around-childbirth-photos

14   'One Day Young: The first few hours of life', Tom Seymour, bbc.com, 3 December 2015. http://www.bbc.com/culture/story/20151201-one-day-young-the-first-few-hours-of-life

15  'One Day Young' interview with Jenny Lewis, Mel Luff, *People of Print*, 9 March 2016. https://www.peopleofprint.com/general/ jenny-lewis-one-day-young-interview/

16  '#birthjusthappened: the photos changing the way we see labour', Catherine Rodie, *Essential Baby*, 31 March 2015. http://www. essentialbaby.com.au/birth/stages-of-labour/birthjusthappened- the-photos-changing-the-way-we-see-labour-20150331-1mbmam

17  '#BirthJustHappened: Post-birth selfies are exactly what women need', Milli Hill, *Telegraph*, 20 March 2015. https://www. telegraph.co.uk/women/mother-tongue/11483462/BirthJustHap- pened-Post-birth-selfies-are-what-women-need.html

18  https://www.birthundisturbed.com/

19  *Childbirth Without Fear*, Grantly Dick-Read, Heinemann Medical Books, 1942. Second edition, Pinter & Martin Ltd, London, 2013

20  https://www.instagram.com/natalielennard/

21  http://birth-media.com/laboring-under-an-illusion/

22  'Private view, public birth: making feminist sense of the new visual culture of childbirth', Lisa Baraitser, *Studies in the Maternal*, vol. 5, issue 2, 2013.
    http://www.research.lancs.ac.uk/portal/en/publications/private- view-public-birth(7e479b47-5da2-40e9-8d22-7ac08067ed1c).html

23  'Quantitative insights into televised birth: a content analysis of *One Born Every Minute*, Sara De Benedictis et al., *Critical Studies in Media Communication*, vol.36, issue 1, 2019. https://www.tand- fonline.com/doi/full/10.1080/15295036.2018.1516046?

24  *A Good Birth, a Safe Birth: Choosing and Having the Childbirth Experience You Want*, Diana Korte, Harvard Common Press (3rd ed.), Boston, 1992

25  'Healthcare professionals' assertions and women's responses during labour: A conversation analytic study of data from *One Born Every Minute*', C. Jackson et al., *Patient Education and Counselling*, vol. 100, issue 3, March 2017. https://www.ncbi.nlm.nih.gov/ pubmed/27769589

26  https://www.birthyouinlove.com/better-antenatal-education/ my-thoughts-on-delivering-babies-with-emma-willis-episode-1/

27    'Men need to better prepare for the "gore" of childbirth', Milli Hill, *Telegraph*, 18 April 2013. https://www.telegraph.co.uk/women/mother-tongue/10003723/Men-need-to-better-prepare-for-the-gore-of-childbirth.html

28    As described in *Recovery: Freedom From Our Addictions*, Russell Brand, Bluebird, London, 2017, and as an edited extract at https://www.whimn.com.au/strength/mind/russell-brand-shares-the-incredibly-personal-story-of-his-daughters-birth/news-story/38a318762ade23224967d4aef714a951

29    https://www.instagram.com/p/Bh7Amsfl_pd/?fbclid=IwAR0dPs-8D1oxcGGtdUZ6CLD2KIBgmbdsHZKZzy9nqvRKAy-tOCdBGUd4W43Gs

30    'So then. Bridget Jones' Baby . . .', Ralph Jones, *Medium*, 23 February 2017. https://medium.com/@OhHiRalphJones/so-then-bridget-jones-baby-6c42efe9066b

31    'Harry Kane, the main thing about giving birth is mother and baby's health', Barbara Ellen, *Guardian*, 11 August 2018. https://www.theguardian.com/commentisfree/2018/aug/11/actually-harry-kane-no-one-cares-how-you-give-birth-as-long-as-the-baby-is-safely-delivered

32    *On Becoming a Mother: Welcoming Your New Baby and Your New Life with Wisdom from Around the World*, Brigid McConville, Oneworld Publications, London, 2014

33    Research carried out by academics at City, University of London, in 2017. https://www.city.ac.uk/news/2017/february/maternal-ptsd-could-affect-up-to-28,000-women-in-the-uk-each-year,-says-new-review?fbclid=IwAR36tuBiTlGGVvF5gZct4MfWtlr-wN5Qc2Z_juzm_a0S9f1OZElAHHlpY_os

34    'The Need to Humanize Birth in Australia', Marsden Wagner, paper presented at the Homebirth Australia Conference, Noosa, Australia, November 2000. https://birthinternational.com/article/birth/fish-cant-see-water/?doing_wp_cron=1550229753.6224200725555419921875

# CHAPTER 7

1    *A Vindication for the Rights of Woman*, Mary Wollstonecraft, 1792

2    http://www.birthrights.org.uk/resources/your-rights/

3    'Maternity care providers' perceptions of women's autonomy and the law', Sue Kruske et al., *BMC Pregnancy and Childbirth*, 4 April 2013. https://bmcpregnancychildbirth.biomedcentral.com/articles/10.1186/1471-2393-13-84

4    https://www.nycourts.gov/ctapps/Decisions/2015/Oct15/179opn15-Decision.pdf

5    http://helpchristinetaylor.blogspot.com/

6    'More and more laws are treating a fetus as a person, and a woman as less of one, as states charge pregnant women with crimes…', *The New York Times* Opinion, 28 December 2018. https://www.nytimes.com/interactive/2018/12/28/opinion/pregnancy-women-pro-life-abortion.html

7    'Should Pregnant Women Be Put in Jail for Drinking?', Jessica Wakeman, Healthline.com, 20 February 2018. https://www.healthline.com/health-news/should-pregnant-women-be-jailed-for-drinking#1

8    'Court of Appeal rules that drinking in pregnancy is not a crime', birthrights.org.uk, 4 December 2014. http://www.birthrights.org.uk/2014/12/court-of-appeal-rules-that-drinking-in-pregnancy-is-not-a-crime/

9    http://hudoc.echr.coe.int/app/conversion/pdf/?Library=-ECHR&id=001-102254&filename=001-102254.pdf

10   http://microbirth.com/freedom-for-birth/

11   *Human Rights in Childbirth,* ed. Hermine Hayes-Klein, Bynkershoek Conference Papers, 2012. http://komora-primalja.hr/datoteke/Human%20Rights%20in%20Childbirth%20Conference%20Papers.pdf

12   Ibid

13   https://www.whiteribbonalliance.org/wp-content/uploads/2017/11/Final_RMC_Charter.pdf

14   'The #matexp lithotomy challenge', Leigh Kendall, *Maternity Experience*, 31 May 2015. http://matexp.org.uk/matexp-and-me/the-matexp-lithotomy-challenge/

15   'Birth Outside the Box – #TheatreChallenge!', Katherine Mabey, All4maternity.com, 3 December 2017. https://www.all4maternity.com/birth-outside-box-theatrechallenge/

16   https://www.supremecourt.uk/decided-cases/docs/UKSC_2013_0136_Judgment.pdf

17   'Montgomery is the belated obituary, not the death knell, of medical paternalism, says Charles Foster', Charles Foster, *New Law Journal*, issue 7647. https://www.newlawjournal.co.uk/content/last-word-consent

18   'Transforming consent in maternity care', report on the October 2017 Birthrights seminar, part of the Sheila Kitzinger Programme, Green Templeton College, Oxford. https://www.gtc.ox.ac.uk/wp-content/uploads/2018/12/Transforming-Consent-Report-Co-branded-Final-April18.pdf

19   https://www.nhs.uk/conditions/consent-to-treatment/capacity/

20   https://www.gov.uk/government/publications/the-nhs-constitution-for-england

21   'Attitudes to sexual consent', Research for the End Violence Against Women Coalition by YouGov, December 2018. https://www.endviolenceagainstwomen.org.uk/wp-content/uploads/1-Attitudes-to-sexual-consent-Research-findings-FINAL.pdf

22   'Dignity in Childbirth', The Dignity Survey 2013: Women's and midwives' experiences of UK maternity care, Birthrights Dignity in Childbirth Forum, 16 October 2013. http://www.birthrights.org.uk/wordpress/wp-content/uploads/2013/10/Birthrights-Dignity-Survey.pdf

23   Unpublished survey

24   'Listening to Mothers III: Pregnancy and Birth', *Report of the Third National U.S. Survey of Women's Childbearing Experiences*, Eugene R. Declercq et al., May 2013. http://transform.childbirthconnection.org/wp-content/uploads/2013/06/LTM-III_Pregnancy-and-Birth.pdf

25   https://mothermayithemovie.com/

26   https://www.birthcompanions.org.uk/

27   'Why America's Black Mothers and Babies Are in a Life-or-Death Crisis', Linda Vallarosa, *The New York Times*, 11 April 2018. https://www.nytimes.com/2018/04/11/magazine/black-mothers-babies-death-maternal-mortality.html

28   'MBRRACE-UK: Saving Lives, Improving Mothers' Care: Lessons learned to inform maternity care from the UK and Ireland Confidential Enquiries into Maternal Deaths and Morbidity 2014–16', Nuffield Department of Population Health, University of Oxford, last updated 31 October 2018. https://www.npeu.ox.ac.uk/mbrrace-uk/reports

29   'Doctors Often Fail to Listen to Black Mothers, Complicating Births, Survey Finds', Fran Kritz, *California Health Report*, 20 September 2018. http://www.calhealthreport.org/2018/09/20/doctors-often-fail-listen-black-mothers-complicating-births-survey-finds/

30   'Dubska ECHR judgment: disappointing but not the last word', Rebecca Schiller, birthrights.org.uk, 15 November 2016. http://www.birthrights.org.uk/2016/11/disappointing-echr-judgment/

31   'Consent and student medics – European Court ruling', birthrights.org.uk, 14 October 2014. http://www.birthrights.org.uk/2014/10/consent-and-student-medics-european-court-ruling/

32   'Jury awards Mountain Brook couple $16 million in case against Brookwood Medical Center', Kent Faulk, al.com, 6 August 2016. https://www.al.com/news/birmingham/index.ssf/2016/08/jury_awards_mountain_brook_cou.html

33   WHO recommendation on respectful maternity care during labour and childbirth, 15 February 2018. https://extranet.who.int/rhl/topics/preconception-pregnancy-childbirth-and-postpartum-care/care-during-childbirth/who-recommendation-respectful-maternity-care-during-labour-and-childbirth

34   https://www.whiteribbonalliance.org/whatwomenwant/

## CHAPTER 8

1    *A Journal of the Plague Year*, Daniel Defoe, Penguin Classics, 2003
2    'A reckoning: the continuing cost of COVID-19', NHS Confederation, 2 September 2021. https://www.nhsconfed.org/sites/default/files/2021-09/A-reckoning-continuing-cost-of-COVID-19.pdf
3    'How is the Covid-19 Crisis Affecting the NHS', Heidi Karjalainen, Economics Observatory, 24 November 2021. https://www.economicsobservatory.com/update-how-is-the-covid-19-crisis-affecting-the-nhs
4    ButNotMaternity.org
5    Petition entitled 'Partners allowed for entirety of labour/birth in ALL hospitals', https://www.change.org/p/partners-allowed-for-entirety-of-labour-birth-in-all-hospitals-butnotmaternity
6    'One fifth of mums giving birth during the pandemic have felt forced to have a vaginal examination in labour', Pregnant Then Screwed, 16 November 2020. https://pregnantthenscrewed.com/press-release-one-fifth-of-mums-giving-birth-during-the-pandemic-have-felt-forced-to-have-a-vaginal-examination-in-labour/
7    'How pregnant women are feeling forced into "violating" vaginal examinations during Covid, *Telegraph*, 20 November 2020
8    Online survey carried out by Positive Birth Movement and Channel Mum in 2016. https://www.positivebirthmovement.org/birth-survey-2016/
9    'Birth characteristics in England and Wales: 2020', Office for National Statistics, 13 January 2022. https://www.ons.gov.uk/peoplepopulationandcommunity/birthsdeathsandmarriages/livebirths/bulletins/birthcharacteristicsinenglandandwales/2020#:
10   'Changes in home births by race and Hispanic origin and state of residence of mother: United States, 2018–2019 and 2019–2020', Elizabeth C.W. Gregory et al., National Vital Statistics Report, Vol. 70, No 15, 9 December 2021. https://www.cdc.gov/nchs/data/nvsr/nvsr70/NVSR70-15.pdf
11   'UK health trusts suspend home birth services as midwives shortage deepens', Hannah Summers, *Observer*, 28 November 2021. https://www.theguardian.com/lifeandstyle/2021/nov/28/

uk-health-trusts-suspend-home-birth-services-midwives-shortage

12  Statistics provided directly from Private Midwives.

13  'Between a rock and a hard place: considering "freebirth during Covid-19", Mari Greenfield et al., *Frontiers in Global Women's Health*, 18 February 2021. https://www.frontiersin.org/articles/10.3389/fgwh.2021.603744/full

14  'Obstetric interventions and pregnancy outcomes during the Covid-19 pandemic in England: A nationwide cohort study', Ipek Gurol-Urganci et al., *Plos Medicine*, 10 January 2022. https://journals.plos.org/plosmedicine/article?id=10.1371/journal.pmed.1003884

15  'Giving birth in a pandemic: Women's birth experiences in England during Covid-19', Ezra Aydin et al., MedRxiv, *BMC Pregnancy and Childbirth*, 6 July 2021. https://www.medrxiv.org/content/10.1101/2021.07.05.21260022v1.full

16  'The mental health crisis of expectant women in the UK: Effects of the Covid-19 pandemic on prenatal mental health, antenatal attachment and social support', Maria Laura Filippetti et al., *BMC Pregnancy and Childbirth*, 26 January 2022. https://bmcpregnancychildbirth.biomedcentral.com/articles/10.1186/s12884-022-04387-7#:

17  'Childbirth during Covid-19 pandemic associated with anxiety, post-traumatic stress symptoms, NIH-supported study suggests', National Institute of Child Health and Human Development', 19 January 2021. https://www.nichd.nih.gov/newsroom/news/011921-childbirth-COVID-19

18  'Mothers forced to give birth alone during Covid pandemic speak of the "trauma" of hospital restrictions', Joe Duggan, *The i*, 19 January 2022. https://inews.co.uk/news/mothers-forced-give-birth-alone-covid-pandemic-hospital-restrictions-1403949

19  'NHS gains just one extra midwife for every 30 trained', Royal College of Midwives, 11 September 2018. https://www.rcm.org.

uk/media-releases/2018/september/nhs-gains-just-one-extra-midwife-for-every-30-trained-new-rcm-report/

20   'Midwives are at breaking point and soon there won't be any left', Faye Brown, *Metro*, 21 November 2021. https://metro.co.uk/2021/11/21/nhs-midwives-are-at-breaking-point-and-soon-there-wont-be-any-left-15633788/

21   'Stem the tide of midwives leaving the profession, RCM tells Downing Street', Royal College of Midwives, 17 February 2022. https://www.rcm.org.uk/media-releases/2022/february/stem-the-tide-of-midwives-leaving-the-profession-rcm-tells-downing-street/

22   'Immediate and essential actions to improve care and safety in maternity services across England', from the Ockenden Review, 30 March 2022. https://www.gov.uk/government/publications/final-report-of-the-ockenden-review/ockenden-review-sum-mary-of-findings-conclusions-and-essential-actions#immedi-ate-and-essential-actions-to-improve-care-and-safety-in-mater-nity-services-across-england

23   'Three hundred babies lost to a fixation on natural births', Shaun Lintern, *The Times*, 26 March 2022. https://www.thetimes.co.uk/article/fatal-nhs-obsession-with-natural-births-nxdsvxn5v

24   UN Women report on 'Covid-19: Rebuilding for resilience'. https://www.unwomen.org/en/hq-complex-page/covid-19-rebuild-ing-for-resilience

25   'Women and the pandemic: Serious damage to work, health and home demands response', Tracy Brower, *Forbes*, 18 April 2021. https://www.forbes.com/sites/tracybrower/2021/04/18/women-and-the-pandemic-serious-damage-to-work-health-and-home-demands-response/?sh=6a6571fb1f49

26   'Pandemic hits mental health of women and young people hardest, study finds', Jon Henley, *Guardian*, 23 November 2021. https://www.theguardian.com/world/2021/nov/23/pandemic-hits-men-tal-health-of-women-and-young-people-hardest-survey-finds

27   'Covid-19 pandemic hits mental health, especially of the young and of women, and widens inequalities', James Banks and Xiaowei

Xu, Institute for Fiscal Studies, 10 June 2020. https://ifs.org.uk/publications/14876

28  'Most Britons cannot name all parts of vulva, survey reveals', Linda Geddes, *Guardian*, 30 May 2021. https://www.theguardian.com/lifeandstyle/2021/may/30/most-britons-cannot-name-parts-vul-va-survey

29  'Almost 50% of women don't know where their cervix or uterus is, nor the purpose of menstruation, study finds', Faima Bakar, *Metro*, 9 November 2020. https://metro.co.uk/2020/11/09/almost-50-of-women-dont-know-where-their-cervix-is-finds-study-13561743/

30  '73% of women still confused about what a vulva is', Rachel Moss, *Huffington Post*, 28 March 2019. https://www.huffingtonpost.co.uk/entry/73-of-women-still-confused-about-what-a-vulva-is-so-heres-the-diagram-you-need_uk_5c9b5970e4b072a7f6022a74

31  'Take the vulva vow', The Eve Appeal. https://eveappeal.org.uk/blog/take-the-vulva-vow/

32  https://www.nhs.uk/conditions/gender-dysphoria/

33  'Sex is binary: Scientists speak up for the empirical reality of biological sex', Fair Play for Women, 14 February 2020. https://fairplayforwomen.com/scientistsspeak/

34  'Sex redefined: The idea of 2 sexes is overly simplistic', Claire Ainsworth, *Nurture* magazine, via *Scientific American*, 22 October 2018. https://www.scientificamerican.com/article/sex-redefined-the-idea-of-2-sexes-is-overly-simplistic1/

35  'Open letter to MANA', Woman-Centred Midwifery, 20 August 2015. https://womancenteredmidwifery.wordpress.com/take-action/

36  'Idealized and Industrialized Labor: Anatomy of a Feminist Controversy', Jane Clare Jones, Hypatia, Vol. 27, No 1, 2012.

37  'Royal Academy apologises to artist Jess de Wahls in transphobia row' BBC News, 23 June 2021. https://www.bbc.co.uk/news/entertainment-arts-57578732

38  https://www.chimamanda.com/news_items/it-is-obscene-a-true-reflection-in-three-parts/

39    'Maya Forstater: Woman discriminated against over trans tweets, tribunal rules', BBC News, 6 July 2022. https://www.bbc.co.uk/news/uk-62061929

40    'Look at the numbers and times: No denying the advantages of Lia Thomas', John Lohn, *Swimming World*, 5 April 2022. https://www.swimmingworldmagazine.com/news/a-look-at-the-numbers-and-times-no-denying-the-advantages-of-lia-thomas/

41    'Effective communication about pregnancy, birth, lactation, breast-feeding and newborn care: The importance of sexed language', Kathleen Gribble et al., *Frontiers in Global Women's Health*, February 2022. https://www.frontiersin.org/articles/10.3389/fgwh.2022.818856/full

42    'Our values. Our vision. Our ambitions', British Pregnancy Advisory Service, September 2021. https://www.bpas.org/media/3550/bpas-advocacy-values-vision-ambitions.pdf

43    BPAS open letter, 15 October 2021. https://www.repropact.com/_files/ugd/680104_359650884f1142cbb1fab37735de590f.pdf

44    With Women's open letter to the BPAS board of trustees and senior management team, https://with-woman.org/2021/10/21/open-letter-to-bpas/

# Index

## ONE PLACE. MANY STORIES

Bold, innovative and
empowering publishing.

FOLLOW US ON:

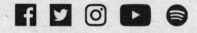

@HQStories